ALTERNATIVE
MEDICINE
O•N•L•I•N•E

ALTERNATIVE
MEDICINE
O·N·L·I·N·E

A Guide to
Natural Remedies
on the Internet

Ralph W. Moss, Ph.D.

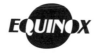

Equinox Press, Inc.
Brooklyn, New York

Copyright © 1997 by Ralph W. Moss

Manufactured in the United States of America by

Equinox Press

144 St. John's Place

Brooklyn, NY 11217

718-636-1679

Typography and design by Movable Type, Inc.

1   3   5   7   9   10   8   6   4   2

Library of Congress Cataloging-in-Publication Data

Moss, Ralph W.
    Alternative medicine online : a guide to natural remedies on the
internet / Ralph W. Moss.
        p.   cm.
    Includes index.
    ISBN 1-881025-10-1 (pbk.)
    1. Alternative medicine – – Computer network resources. 2. Internet
(Computer network)   I. Title.
R733.M68   1997   97-22650
025.06'61 – – dc21   CIP

TABLE OF CONTENTS

PREFACE:
OBSESSION

In my fifth decade, when a man
is supposed to be past all likelihood of
childish infatuation, I fell head over heels in love.
Deep yearnings arouse me and we spend long hours
together in intimate hand and eye contact.

This obsession occupies half of my waking hours. It even has invaded and disturbed my dreams, as I pursue combinations and positions unattainable in the physical world.

My friends are laughing at me, and I know I am the object of whispers. They don't know the half of it, either. Oddest of all, the object of my affection is neither woman, man, boy, girl, pig nor dog. I am not sure it can even be classified as a material thing. I am writing a book about it, but I don't even know what it is. I don't think anyone can really define it, although the most insightful world leaders glimpse in this infatuation the future of the human race. It is of course the Internet. And for me, as for thousands of others, it has truly become a Web without a Weaver, a Web into which we have inextricably fallen without any possibility of escape.

Just out of curiosity, I downloaded a log of some of my recent Internet sessions. In fact, I would reprint last month's log for you here, so you could gauge the extent of my obsession for yourself—

except that it takes up 29 pages, single spaced. But here's the record of a fairly typical work day:

6:58 AM	Connection at 28800 bps.	11:54 AM	Connection terminated.
7:44 AM	Connection terminated.	12:30 PM	Connection at 28800 bps.
8:34 AM	Connection at 28800 bps.	1:03 PM	Connection terminated.
8:49 AM	Connection terminated.	1:13 PM	Connection at 28800 bps.
9:19 AM	Connection at 26400 bps.	1:57 PM	Connection terminated.
10:32 AM	Connection terminated.	3:42 PM	Connection at 26400 bps.
11:07 AM	Connection at 28800 bps.	4:28 PM	Connection terminated.

As you can see, in the course of ten hours I logged on seven times and spent half the day—about five hours time, all told—on the World Wide Web. And I didn't just leave the clock running, the way some people do. That's actual working time you are looking at. I would say that qualifies as an obsession, wouldn't you?

Amazingly, a few years ago I— and most of the rest of us — had never even heard of the Internet. I had worked a lot on Compuserve and the other online services, however. (I even wrote an article in 1992 in which I described myself as a "Compu-slave.") Then, in November, 1993 I was asked to take part in an exploratory visit from the Office of Alternative Medicine (OAM) to the home of the pioneering Sunsite at the University of North Carolina. I and a team of OAM staff members and advisors flew into Chapel Hill, then sat through a day of presentations about Unix. (At first, I thought I had accidentally walked in on a lecture on Renaissance music.)

Sunsite (http://sunsite.unc.edu/) was and is considered one of the premiere Internet locations. It contains a vast array of texts on numerous topics, one of which was alternative medicine. The irony of that day was that these experts couldn't make the Internet connection to the space-age auditorium in which we sat. So the Internet still remained an abstraction for us. I and the other OAM emissaries left Chapel Hill almost as confused as when we had arrived, but with admiration for the enormous enthusiasm generated by the concept of world-wide computer linkage. Dozing on the plane coming home, I began to form in my mind an image of the Internet as a new stage in evolution, an electronic nervous system linking the "brain cells" of individuals, as expressed through their computers. It is a vision that hasn't left me.

This book brings together my two great obsessions. Since Vice President Gore's speech in the 1992 Vice Presidential debates, Internet has been one of the buzzwords of the new age. But few people realize how it intersects with that other hot topic, "alternative medicine." America's love affair with far-out medicine dates from around the same time. Oddly, despite hundreds of books on each of these topics, this is the first book I am aware of that brings both of these worlds together.

I realize that some people have difficulty understanding the appeal of alternative medicine. They think it is a fad, which will run its course. I don't think so. If it is a fad, it is showing unusual staying power. A survey of "ordinary" patients showed that interest in alternative and complementary treatments continues to grow apace. The study in question surveyed patients enrolled in four family practices in the western United States. It was published by Nancy C. Elder, MD of the Oregon Health Sciences University, in an orthodox journal, the March/April 1997 edition of the Archives of Family Medicine.

The article reveals that 50 percent of these typical American patients either had used or were currently using acupuncture, chiropractic, homeopathy, other forms of alternative medicine. This usage is up from the benchmark article which showed that one-third used such treatments just a few years before, as reported in the New England Journal of Medicine in 1993. It is interesting that half of the Oregon patients who were using alternatives had not informed their physicians of this fact. It would not surprise me if many of them also found out about such treatments on the Internet, which has become a vast meeting place for people feeling disenfranchised by the medical establishment. How do I know about all this? I read about it on the Net.

Hopefully, this book can aid people in making medical choices. Clearly, there is a lot of medical foolishness out there on the Net. As with anything, exposure to many points of view, excellently presented, can make wise consumers out of casual surfers.

My criteria for inclusion in this book. How did I make the decision to include a site in this book? Since there are so many potential sites, you would think that I would have well defined criteria for choosing and including sites in my book. However, being left-handed and right-brained, I more or less let whimsy guide me. I looked in thousands of out-of-the-way places but few of them made the cut. And while I toyed with the idea of setting up some rating schema, in the end it was my own personal predilections that ruled. Did the site amuse me? Did it make me want to bookmark it and come back?

This is a personal and subjective selection. Some people may be disappointed that a favorite place has been overlooked or omitted, but that is inevitable. Also, I have not made a great effort to systematically cover the whole panoply of human diseases or of alternative methods currently in use. Sometimes I wanted very much to cover a particular topic, but could not find a site to my liking. Thus, if I have inadvertently left holes in this impressionistic picture, I would appreciate leads email-ed to mail@ralphmoss.com. I will consider your suggestions for future editions.

That said, I did evolve some criteria—call them pet peeves, if you like—which substituted for rules. I would like to share them with you:

Spelling and grammar. The editor of the Journal of the American Medical Association has called the Internet "the world's largest vanity press." So if the Internet is to be taken seriously as publishing, it should behave like a responsible medium. To me, that means, at the very least, a minimum of typos.

In just one brief online session, I came across the following errors: "Patterns can be seen through a automated microscope." A automated microscope? I couldn't go one click further as an imaginary cane appeared and yanked this contender off my mental stage.

Or how about this one: "More pages are comming soon." Or this: "Nurses, For More Indepenents...." The same site offered readers a selection of "Classified adds." Call me a snob, but if you can't spell a two-letter word or have such a tin ear that you can actually say "a automated" anything, how can we trust anything else you might say?

Aesthetics. I am not a professional HTML maven. Yet I manage to write clear and simple pages and upload them to my own site. I am therefore intolerant of pages that assault and offend the eye or ear. I reject as a barbarity all pages written in yellow type on a white background. I object to pages that are written entirely in large headline type, especially those selling herbs originating anywhere on the other side of the International Date Line. I can't abide pages in which every line is written in a different rainbow color. They don't make me euphoric; they make me clinically depressed.

And, incidentally, I reject all pages whose fraud is palpable. I don't just mean bogus claims for cancer cures. I mean people who fiddle with the odometer to show over 1,250,000 hits in under ten days of operation, as one pathetic site recently did.

Commercialism. I am not a purist on the question of salesmanship on the Net. Overall, I'm glad people can sell stuff online. Certainly, many excellent health sites advertise valuable books, tapes or consulting services. But sites that are overwhelmingly commercial generally don't hold my interest. I gravitate towards content-rich sites, where experts foolishly give away what they know.

An example you will read about is Michael Moore's herbal site (http://chili.rt66.com/hrbmoore/HOMEPAGE/HomePage.html). Moore reprints many of his books and lecture notes right at the site. As a result, this is one of the best visited independent health sites on the Internet, with over 1,000 hits per day. I would like to believe this generosity will be rewarded, in Heaven if not on Earth. Experts say that putting your books on the Internet increases physical book sales or seminar enrollments. I hope this is true. In any case, Michael is certainly helping a lot of folks, and improving the quality and scope of information available.

By contrast, I bristle at those slick sites that try to nickel and dime you to death for every bit of information they stingily dole out. One free "news" clipping service I subscribe to tries to hit me up for an additional $1.00 or $4.00 for every article I choose to download. I hate to pay for such info when I can probably find it elsewhere for nothing. I mean, for $4.00 I could get a double decaf latte macchiato at Starbucks. Consequently, you won't find too many of those pay-per-view sites in this book, either.

Promises. I don't like sites that promise more than they deliver. For example, I tend to shun grandiose directories of medical practitioners. A lot of people had the bright idea to create such directories and then charge practitioners for the privilege of being listed therein. By and large, it hasn't happened and so most of these helpful directories are wishful thinking. They are usually elaborate shells. One I looked at had no practitioners at all in New York City—no acupuncturists, no homeopaths, no nothing. Not a good sign. Others have obviously incorporated the membership lists of a few organizations, but are lacking live participants.

Another pet peeve: I can't stand those clever little "under construction" signs, with their stick figures digging holes. Everything on the Internet should be part of an ongoing growth process.

Interest level. The Net in my view should be odd, zany, fascinating. Yet some sites are just like slick brochures you pick up in your doctor's office. Here's my bias: I tend to shun Authoritative Sites put together by committees and instead I gravitate towards wacky ones. I can only hope that no one will fall seriously ill because they were waylayed by medical Alchemists when they were trying to find the AMA. Where else but on the Internet are you likely to learn about Yogic flying, pulse diagnosis, urine therapy, and the like? This is the stuff that fills up the hard drives of online quackbusters. I'm big on documentation but on the other hand I enjoy the anarchic nature of the Net. Such sites amuse me and broaden my horizons.

Individualism. In a related vein, one of the things I celebrate is the possibility of rugged individualism on the electronic frontier. (I could get a job as Al Gore's speechwriter!) It astonishes and delights me to see how one individual, living in a trailer in rural California, can create a Website that dwarfs in importance and sometimes even size those of multi-billion dollar institutions. I am thinking particularly of Sister Mary Elizabeth who single-handedly created the most comprehensive site on AIDS on the Net (http://www.aegis.com/). But the same applies to an excellent cancer site, authored by a patient, Steve Dunn (http://cancerguide.org). A Swedish teacher, Leif Hedegard, put together the best site, in my opinion, on the question of dental amalgams, pro and con, which could serve as a model for dealing in a responsible way with medical controversies (http://www.algonet.se/~leif/AmFAQigr.html). Yet, it was only as this book was going to press that the OAM finally posted its own Web site, after four years of effort (http://altmed.od.nih.gov).

Helpfulness. I also sought out sites that could shed new light on old problems. It is said, for instance, that 100,000,000 Americans are now living with chronic illnesses of some sort. Many of these people have sad tales to tell: of being treated in a dismissive way by their doctors ("It's all in your head"), given dangerous and/or ineffective drugs, or told they have to live with the problem.

I get especially excited when I find a site that offers hope for persistent medical problems. For example, I got really charged up when I discovered the Buteyko treatment for asthma (http://www.gil.com.au/~pathein/video/method.html). This is a growing movement in the Commonwealth countries, but virtually unknown elsewhere. I emailed the reference to a friend of mine who suffers from asthma and she is exploring the treatment now. This is the Internet at its best. Sure, it may not pan out for her. But at least it gives her the feeling that there are possible solutions, other than an "addiction" to her inhalers.

Internationalism. I have always disliked the narrow chauvinism of some American scientists. I once debated an oncologist on television in Indianapolis. He was a nice enough fellow, but when I brought up some Russian studies, he stared into the camera and declared, "I don't believe any study not done in the US." An NIH draft dismissed another European treatment on the grounds that it provided "no controlled trials that would meet the requirements of a scientific study in the United States." I wrote the author, "What exactly are the 'requirements' of a scientific study? That it be done in the US?" American medicine is sometimes blind to much of what happens outside its borders. But three quarters of the people in the world depend on what we call "alternative medicine" as their primary form of health care. For practical reasons, I have limited my discussion to English-language sites. And luckily for us Anglophones most of the Net is in English. But I cherish the internationalism of the Net and am happy to include sites from various nations, countries and climes.

Accuracy. Of course, I am interested in accuracy, especially in regard to medicine. As Mark Twain perspicaciously said, "Be careful about reading health books. You may die of a misprint."

But while some things are a matter of fact, most "facts" are a matter of opinion and interpretation. At this moment we are in the midst of a vast debate on the value of mammography for women in their forties. Speak to the American Cancer Society and its efficacy is a matter of fact. Speak to other experts and it is much less certain. (Still others regard them as positively dangerous.) Beware of "facts" which brook no opposition. If we don't allow room for unorthodox ideas, we are unlikely to make great breakthroughs. And in most areas of medicine great breakthroughs are needed.

The American Medical Association, not surprisingly, has a different take. They are into authority. In their April 16, 1997 Journal they sound the alarm about burgeoning quackery on the Internet. "Information on the Internet is subject to the same rules and regulations as conversation at a bar," sneered editor George D. Lundberg, MD. "It may be very valid; it may be utter trash."

In the same vein, Dr. Dave Jenkinson of the University of Pittsburgh demanded to know, "'Who's putting it on?' If someone is coming up with a position, do they have the research to back it up, and is the research credible?"

Simultaneously, it was announced that the federal government was moving into action. It has organized its Web-based materials to make them easier to search. A new site called www.healthfinder.gov was launched April 15—an inauspicious day for the government to spend anyone's tax dollars—and will offer links to more than 800 consumer health Web sites including 300 federal sites.

Of course, the doyens of conventional medicine say they have no intention of "censoring" the Net. But given their history, is it Web-induced paranoia to find their disclaimers less than reassuring?

Web focus. This book is called "Alternative Medicine Online" but that is not exactly accurate. For what the book is primarily about is the Internet, and particularly the World Wide Web. Thus, I do not deal with online services like America Online (AOL).There are plenty of guides to that world, and surfing the Web through AOL has always seemed less than satisfying to me.

I also do not deal at length with another aspect of the online world that is important to some people. I am referring to discussion groups, called Listservs or Newsgroups. There are thousands of such groups on the Net. Each of these is a collection of articles (essentially, email messages) which are theoretically related to a particular topic. You can subscribe to (join) a newsgroup discussion on any topic that interests you.

Access. Studies show that as of mid-1996, there were 37 million people in the US and Canada, over the age of 16, who had access to the Internet; and 17.6 million of these were actively using the World Wide Web. It is also estimated that there will be over 200 million people on the Web by the year 2005. These facts have enormous implications for the future of medicine.

The most revolutionary element in medicine has always been the patient's access to medical information. A long time ago Francis Bacon said "Knowledge is Power." One could argue that it has always been conventional doctors' virtual monopoly of knowledge combined with control of the sources of public information, that has given them their power as the preeminent "sovereign profession."

The proliferation of health books written by lay people began to equalize the equation. The Internet enormously accelerates that change. As Dr. Lundberg remarks, everyone is his own publisher these days. The AMA's site is not intrinsically more believable than the guy with the improbable cure. In fact, if the fringe guy has a particular talent for Web design, his site may be far more compelling and interesting than the establishment's.

Although some in conventional medicine don't realize it yet, the Internet has tilted the balance in the doctor-patient relationship. Doctors are getting used to patients showing up with downloads from the Net, some of them even printed out in color. Their patients are becoming instant experts, and know more about some topics than they do.

Some doctors have responded in a wonderful way, by throwing themselves into the Net, participating in debates, and testing their ideas against those of skeptical medical consumers. Prostate Pointers (http://rattler.cameron.edu/prostate/) is one such site where doctors match their wits with savvy patients. Andrew Weil and Deepak Chopra's sites also fit this description. It is a fertile and exciting mixture.

Other health professionals are resisting the change. In either case, all of us involved in the search for health have been handed an amazing tool for exploring not just conventional knowledge but a vast range of options. Like it or not, this is the fruit of humanity's fertile imagination and genius. Ignorance is no longer necessary for any of us. Medical dogma and medical folly are both now exposed to public view. Let the chips fall where they may.

It is my hope that this book will enlighten and entertain you and contribute to a better understanding of the full scope of all your medical choices.   —R.W.M.

ACAM

http://www.acam.org

The American College for Advancement in Medicine (ACAM)
is a non-profit alternative medicine society dedicated to
educating physicians on the latest findings as well as emerging
procedures in preventive/nutritional medicine.

ACAM started out as a society promoting a procedure called 'chelation therapy.' It has grown considerably and its goals are now not only to improve physicians' skills, knowledge, and diagnostic procedures, but also to develop awareness in the public at large of alternative methods of medical treatment.

Specific information about ACAM's programs and philosophy are located in its Web pages. Unlike some medical organizations, ACAM maintains a vibrant and very up-to-date site. There are also membership applications and information about their forthcoming conferences and meetings.

I addressed the group in 1978, when they had "Medical Preventics" in their name. I went back ten years later and was amazed at their growth and prosperity. As stated, ACAM has been closely associated with the use of chelation therapy, which is a technique for "cleaning out" clogged arteries through the use of a non-toxic substance called EDTA. I will not attempt to pass judgment on this controversy. As I understand it, there have been numerous studies showing favorable results, but no large-scale controlled clinical trial has yet been performed. But if you have been diagnosed with coronary artery, circulatory or cardiac diseases of any kind you should at the very least know something about chelation.

This is probably the most authoritative group to discuss the topic. Look for their excellent position paper on this topic (www. acam.org/pospaper.html).

Their position, not surprisingly, is

"...that a more than sufficient quantum of evidence exists to support the use of EDTA chelation therapy as a safe and efficacious treatment modality and, thus, licensed physicians utilizing this therapy should not be impeded in their use of it with their patients."

This is different than what you will hear from your average doc, but then again if your average doc agrees with this s/he should probably be in ACAM. This site also provides a tightly reasoned, fact-filled defense of medical freedom of choice. I intend to bookmark this and return to it many times. Intelligent defenses of this position are difficult to come by, and so a visit is worthwhile.

They even have their own medical journal, the Journal of Advancement in Medicine. Its articles tend to be both provocative and clearly written. For example, the Winter of 1996 issue contained an illuminating article on the benefits of licorice. Many readers will be surprised to find out that this "candy" can have important therapeutic effects.

ACUPUNCTURE

http://www.acupuncture.com/

*"You've got options.
All I really want to do is remind you
that suffering need not be one of them."*

A serene mountain. A quotation from the Tao. "Simply click on the magic words to be transported to the topic of your interest" reads the caption to this excellent site. Welcome to the mysterious world of Eastern medicine, Internet edition.

This is a well visited site and its popularity is well deserved. (They report 62,250 "hits" in the first 10 weeks of 1997.) The reasons for this popularity include the superior aesthetics of their site, the depth of its information, and—not least of all—the sly humor of Webmaster Al Stone.

Every medical site should contain a disclaimer of some sort. (Some consider that the very hallmark of maturity.)

Stone manages to turn a legal department requirement into a philosophical statement: "Take no credit, take no blame. The makers of Acupuncture.com...take no responsibility for the things you may do with this information. We remind you that a little medical knowledge is a dangerous thing and we hope that you will act responsibly with the information you receive on these, and related pages."

I pondered the line "Take no credit, take no blame." It's a nice attitude. If you get benefit from the information provided they don't want the credit for providing it. But neither do they want the blame if something goes wrong.

From the moment you take off your shoes and step onto their turf, you understand that this is no ordinary site. A deep philosophical purpose suffuses their effort. That is why their popularity is heartening and probably why they have won all sorts of awards, been NetGuide's Site of the Day, the "Ask Dr. Weil" Site of the Day, etc.

The depth of information provided here is staggering. Under the Acupuncture heading alone, I counted 22 subheadings. And that is just part of the site. Also, the aesthetics are pleasing. The acupuncture section begins with a beautiful Chinese painting of flowers, gold and needles—a pictorial representation of acupuncture itself.
"For those who read these pages, we're sure you'll
discover that acupuncture is more than just needles, it
is gold," they write.

I'm not sure what it means, but it sounds lovely. Here are some of the other topics covered:

Herbology • Qi Gong • Chinese Nutrition • Tui Na and Chinese Massage • Diagnosis

All in all, there are treasures here. There is, for instance, a translation of a Korean essay from a person named Hun Young Cho, written in 1934, entitled "The Duty of Oriental and Western Medicine." Cho practiced both types of medicine and writes about them eloquently. I found it very thought-provoking. When I discovered a small temporal discrepancy in the article, I emailed Webmaster Stone about it and promptly received back a gracious reply, with an explanation and the promise of a correction. That is impressive. Too many sites are simply put up there and forgotten for months at a time. Most of the outstanding sites are maintained by compulsives who are constantly tinkering with their form and content.

Acupuncture.com site is also valuable as an introduction to the general topic of alternative medicine. Let's face it: if it weren't for the wonderful attitude of the Chinese people, it is doubtful that this field would have progressed as quickly as it has done in the West.

We know that a lot of people use such treatments. But what is the satisfaction rate? That will determine whether or not it is a fad or a permanent part of the landscape. According to Ted Kaptchuk, OMD, of Beth Israel Deaconess Medical Center in Boston, the satisfaction rate with alternative medicine tends to be around 80 percent. But the folks at this site went out and did a survey of users of acupuncture in particular. What did patients think they had derived from it? Here are some of the results:

91.5% reported "disappearance" or "improvement" of symptoms after acupuncture treatment.

84% said they see their medical doctors less.

79% said they use fewer prescription drugs.

70% of those to whom surgery had been recommended said they avoided it.

This data seems to have been carefully collected. No wonder conventional doctors are getting worried! The overwhelming majority of those who try acupuncture seem to like it. Very much. (As I was evaluating this site, by coincidence, I spent time with an elderly lady who told me that she suffered from headaches for 30 years before she tried acupuncture, and within six months they were completely gone. Placebo? Who knows and who cares, with results like that?)

But this is a very practical site as well. With information on specific conditions, it also provides access to practitioners and other providers of acupuncture-related supplies.

Some of the situations that may be helped by acupuncture include the following:

Varicose Veins • Gynecological problems • Pre-menstrual Syndrome • Infertility • Irritable Bowel Syndrome • Arthritis • Carpal Tunnel Syndrome • Drug, Alcohol, Nicotine Addictions

You will need to check your Western preconceptions at the door when you enter the world of acupuncture.com. Thus, in discussing menopause here is Webmaster Al Stone's comments:

> "Traditional Chinese Medicine approaches Menopause as a variety of syndromes. All of them have been successfully treated by acupuncture and herbal medicine. The most typical cause for the symptoms associated with menopause is the slowing of the flow of "Yin." When applied to the health of the physical body, this is the Chinese concept of the hydration or the cooling system within the body...."

I can just see a conventional Western doctor throwing up her hands at this description, or just throwing up. However, given the high rate of success and satisfaction with acupuncture, and the low degree of risk and cost, one might just try this approach, especially if other approaches seem too risky, expensive or invasive.

And there is more. Odd stuff. Have you ever thought about the "smell" of AIDS, for instance. "Smell" in this instance, they explain, is not an olfactory sensation. Webmaster Stone writes:

"I'm not referring to the smells that give the practitioner diagnostic information, but an ineffable cloud that hangs over a patient's life that the practitioner cannot fail to address, and that is the fear of death."

In addition, there are detailed discussions that are aimed primarily at practitioners who treat a wide variety of conditions.

Each essay links you to information about the author, including his or her email address and phone numbers. Contrast this to the situation of the poor person who suffers from one of the above conditions and has access to no other information than what his regular doctor chooses to give him. The Internet is the world in Technicolor.

AEGIS: AIDS EDUCATION

http://www.aegis.com/

This is one of the great success stories of the Internet.
While government agencies dithered,
a single individual created the world's largest source
of information for the health consumer on this difficult topic.

I love this site! It was created in 1990—prehistory as far as the Web is concerned—and is still maintained by Sister Mary Elizabeth, an Episcopal nun (a member of the Sisters of St. Elizabeth of Hungary order). Sister Mary Elizabeth, who has taken a vow of voluntary poverty, lives in a mobile home in the charming old mission town of San Juan Capistrano.

At her wonderful site you can of course glimpse the incredible capacity of the Internet to organize and deliver huge amounts of valuable information in an easy-to-access form. And it also demonstrates the Net's power to make individuals important again in the world of publishing. It can give new meaning to lives.

This one-woman effort is now the largest HIV knowledge base in the entire world. It makes available 3.2 GB ("gigs," i.e., 3,200 "megs") of medical information in over 360,000 documents. In addition, it is all fully indexed and searchable. The site is maintained in part by a grant from a manufacturer of an anti-HIV drug, which is a very wise goodwill investment on their part, but it is still mainly the work of so-called "ordinary" individuals, doing extraordinary things.

This site also contains some features that we would love to see on other sites. There is, for example, a summary of the day's news about AIDS. On the day we looked, there were nine new stories from The New York Times, The Washington Post and USA Today. There were also back issues of this service dating to the first of the year. What an incredible service if you are closely following developments in this particular field, as many people are.

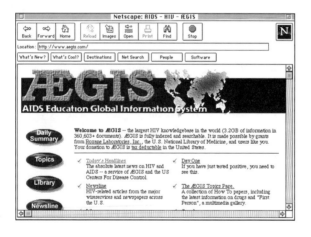

There are very practical items. I found especially excellent (and moving) Wynn Wagner's essay, "Day One." with his four pointers for surviving HIV.

An excellent site.

AESCLEPIUS

http://www.hol.gr/nuclear/public.htm

The Greek Site for Medical and Health Related Information, Resources and Support

This is a very important, if little known, site. While not technically "alternative medicine" (it originates from a radiology department somewhere in Greece), it provides the ammunition for a withering critique of current medical and hygienic practices.

The site is another non-profit endeavor by a dedicated individual. This one is a medical doctor, Costas Giannakenas MD. He has provided a real public service by bringing together a generous selection of articles on a number of public controversies. Some of these are the kind of things you hear fleetingly on the car radio and then, before you focus your attention, they are on to the baseball scores. For me, some of these issues were real eye-openers and I appreciated the possibility the Net gave me to study them at my leisure, seek out opposing positions, and come to some tentative conclusions.

Some of the topics dealt with here:

Aspartame: Is this artificial sweetener dangerous? If you think it is simply impossible that something so popular (over one billion dollars in sales worldwide since 1995) could be deadly, then you need to check out this site. Read the comments of Dr. Erik Millstone of England's University of Sussex, entitled, "Fresh doubts about aspartame's safety." You may be switching to sugar, honey, or maple syrup pretty soon. Did you know that there are ostensibly sane people who call diet drinks "Gulf War Syndrome in a can."

Most ominously, did you know that aspartame is suspected by some as a cause of brain cancer? Or that others talk about a link between Grave's Disease, "dry eyes," and even blindness and the use of this product?! Well, Dr. Giannakenas does come from the part of the world that also gave us Cassandra. But is there some factual basis to his concerns? I think it is worth considering.

Synthetic Genetically-Engineered Bio-Tech Foods: US scientists, with the FDA's blessings, have been fiddling with the food supply. Do such foods pose serious health risks? Did you know that some Europeans are so alarmed over 'genetic soybeans' and the like that they are protesting and cancelling orders for US soybeans? Did you know that some of these protests have been in the nude? (Pictures at eleven.)

Bottle Baby Disease: "...their babies lay, malnourished, dehydrated, sick from Bottle Baby Disease. It doesn't need to happen." Yikes! What is Baby Bottle Disease? Sound crazy? Then read "Baby Milk Powder—is any of it safe?" and articles on Nestle's alleged "cover-up" in Australia.

Bovine Spongiform Encephalopathy and Creutzfeldt-Jakob disease: The establishment is always railing about how the Internet has become a rumor mill. But "mad cow disease" was one of those paranoid Net rumors that turned out to be true. Even the august British Journal of Medicine is now sounding the alarm (and, gloriously, three of their full text articles are given here). I would rate this tops in the "mad cow disease" Website category. And, if you weren't paranoid enough, read how the FDA's approval of a synthetic growth hormone might hasten the spread of mad cow disease around the world.

rBGH (Recombinant Bovine Growth Hormone): Another "high tech nightmare" story. But read about the lawsuit that was filed against the FDA over this controversial agent.

Monosodium Glutamate: An old war horse of a controversy. (I have been assured by several restaurateurs that, regardless of what they say, all Chinese restaurants add MSG to their soups.) Read the collected reports of adverse reactions to MSG. They'll make your head spin.

In addition, The Aesclepius Public Page reprints the complete carcinogen list from the International Agency for Research on Cancer (IARC) of the World Health Organization. This is more inclusive, and therefore less reassuring, than the pro-industry pap that emanates from some big US health agencies.

Electromagnetic Pollution: Here's another one. Is it true that exposure to low level electromagnetic radiation from power lines, electric blankets, video display terminals (VDTs) or even some electric clocks at the head of your bed can cause cancer, birth defects, miscarriages, and other health problems?

My one cavil is that the doctor does not update his site often enough. The last time I checked, his "news" was already six months' old. Nonetheless, it is a unique and valuable service, which deserves wider attention.

AGING RESEARCH

http://www.hookup.net/mall/aging/agesit59.html

Amidst all the ludicrous claims for fountains of youth,
there may be some scientifically valid ways to reverse some
of the effects of aging. But there is a scary aspect to this, too.
People are so desperate to reclaim their youth
that they will submit to almost anything to attain it.

Let me give you my prejudices. Of course, I don't relish getting old. But many of the 'treatments' that people take for this 'condition' scare me. I don't want to fool around with my hormones. I have friends who take melatonin, DHEA, and a host of chemical compounds, and all claim miraculous benefits. I would urge caution: we don't know much about the long-term effects of many of these substances.

That said, I do find the scientific aspect of this quest fascinating. So here is a responsible site that does not seem to be promoting any particular product, but providing researchers and the general public with state-of-the-art information on life prolongation.

Their site reads: "Welcome to the Aging Research Centre (ARC). We are dedicated to providing a service that allows researchers in this field to find information that is related to the study of the aging process. We also endeavor to introduce this field to laymen who would like to know more about the research that is being conducted in this field." Fair enough.

There are scientific articles on cloning, some Real Audio programs on aging, as well as archived Newsgroup discussions. You will find, amidst announcements of meetings of the lively "Cell Death Society" ("pizza will be served") such gems as this bit of scientific free verse:

Clinicians think that they are physiologists;
Physiologists think that they are anatomists;
Anatomists think that they are cell biologists;
Cell biologists think that they are biochemists;
Biochemists think that they are molecular biologists;
Molecular biologists think that they are God;
and what about God?
Well, God does not think !!!

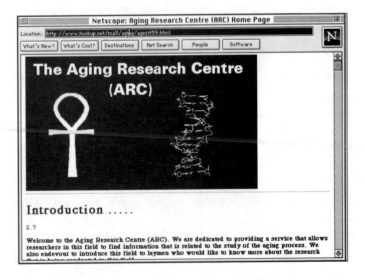

AIDS

http://www.virusmyth.com/aids/

This is a site that gives full exposure to the idea that the HIV virus may not be the cause of the disease known as AIDS. It is a deserving site that is little known or visited.

If you want to learn the orthodox view of AIDS as a viral infection there are numerous sites you can consult. (AEGIS has many such links.) This site offers a disturbing and conflicting view.

Let me say, right off, that this is a clunky site. When you first log on you think there's a problem with your computer. You have to scroll down the page to even find the index. They seriously need a makeover. Also, when I last checked, the site hadn't been updated in almost six months—not a good sign.

I know I will offend some people, for whom HIV is a religion, but I think these ideas deserve an airing. Here's what they say:

"Is HIV really the cause of AIDS? A growing group of bio-medical scientists claim the cause of AIDS is still unknown. These heretics do not believe in a lethal AIDS-virus. They claim that the virus is indeed harmless. AIDS is also not sexually transmitted; it probably has toxic causes, they say. People die because they are poisoned to death by antiviral drugs. These skeptics say that the AIDS virus has never really been isolated, and the AIDS tests are worthless...This website tells you their story."

If you have heard all this before, you can probably skip this site and not disturb yourself further. But if this is news to you, you definitely will want to study the arguments and discuss them with medically oriented friends.

The site itself contains more than 200 pages, with 150 separate articles.

The "Controversy" section rolls out the stars of the presentation here—Nobel Prize winners Kary Mullis and Walter Gilbert, Prof. Harry Rubin of UC Berkeley, etc. Some of the statements by these "heavy weights" might surprise you. They did me, and I thought I was familiar with the terms of the debate.

For instance, how about this one attributed to Dr. Bernard Forscher, former editor of the prestigious Proceedings of the (US) National Academy of Sciences:
> "The HIV hypothesis ranks with the 'bad air' theory for malaria and the 'bacterial infection' theory of beriberi and pellagra [caused by nutritional deficiencies]. It is a hoax that became a scam."

Whoa! Did he really say that? I found particularly fascinating the argument of Dr. Root-Bernstein on the lack of prevalence of AIDS among non-drug-using prostitutes. Turns out that prostitutes in many countries are not dying of AIDS at the rate people predicted. Curious. I'm sure there's a good rebuttal argument, but Root-Bernstein makes a good case for his point of view. You may start to have doubts that HIV is the definitive, single, and solitary cause of the AIDS phenomenon.

ALEXANDER TECHNIQUE

http://www.pavilion.co.uk/stat/welcome.html

**One of the ways in which alternative medicine
has influenced show business and thereby the world
is through the Alexander technique.**

Over the course of a lifetime, F. Matthias Alexander (1869-1955), developed a system of what he called "postural reintegration." He said this could relieve pain and stress by restoring to the body a balanced, regenerative, natural poise. He wrote several books, including the provocatively titled, "The Use of the Self."

It is said that the Alexander technique can be used by almost anybody who wants to restore and maintain a healthy, alert disposition. Over the years it has been especially appreciated by musicians, dancers, and all people who do physically repetitive work. Athletes learn the technique to improve their coordination and general sense of well being.

Illnesses Treated: The Alexander Technique is said to help correct the underlying causes of back pain, neck and shoulder tension, other stress-related illnesses, as well as breathing disorders and fatigue—wherever the misuse or the loss of poise is considered a contributory factor to disease.

What this site says:

> "The Alexander Technique can add a new dimension of awareness, well-being and creativity to most peoples' lives. Because it is concerned with the quality of movement the Technique can benefit anybody with the interest to pursue it."

According to his contemporary, playwright George Bernard Shaw, "Alexander established not only the beginning of a far reaching science of the apparently involuntary movements we call reflexes, but a technique of connection (i.e. integration) and self control which forms a substantial addition to our very slender resources in personal education." John Dewey, another admirer, contributed the preface to his main book. Yet Alexander himself had no medical training. Instead, he was a Shakespearean actor from Australia, trying to solve his own health problems.

Another admirer, Aldous Huxley, wrote that "The Alexander Technique gives all the things we have been looking for....We cannot ask more from any system, nor, if we seriously desire to alter human beings in a desirable direction, can we ask any less." Whoa! High praise indeed from the author of the dystopian and dyspeptic classic, Brave New World.

I don't know much more about Alexander than what I learned at this and similar sites. However, it resonated for me. I am impressed by how wonderful the posture of healthy children is. Yet by the time they are teenagers, they frequently slouch and look uncomfortable in their own skins. If you sit on a bench sometime and watch adults passing on the street, it is like a walking encyclopedia of postural problems.

I am not pointing fingers here: as I write this, sitting at my terminal, I am twisted up into the shape of a pretzel.

The Alexander Technique claims to be able to restore us adults to our natural birthright of good posture.

> "When the natural subconscious mechanisms for balance and posture are disturbed by habitual misuse or injury the standard of our physical and mental functioning can be adversely affected."

That sounds true. "However," he warns, "the appropriate muscular activity for posture is not something we can regain by simply trying harder. It involves 'automatic' reflex responses that, when working well, appear to support the body almost without effort." Breathing and speaking are said to become easier; movement becomes freer, lighter and more enjoyable.

What makes the Alexander Technique so interesting is that it is not only an alternative treatment, it is sort of an "alternative problem," as well, in the sense that conventional medicine does not even recognize bad posture as a condition that forms the prelude to serious bodily and spiritual harm. Clearly, Mr. Alexander was working from a different perspective. Yet the results seem to justify the effort and expense of pursuing this course of bodily re-education.

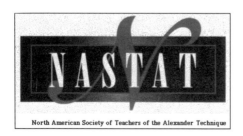

North American Society of Teachers of the Alexander Technique

What we have described is the UK site. While it won't win any design awards, it does a good job of coordinating the various Alexandrian sites on the Internet. What is hinted at in the above GBS quote, however, is that Alexander was more than just a good posture teacher. He had a capital-P Philosophy. Do I sense the slight odor of incense among his disciples? It wouldn't be the first time.

However, if you need a guru, I guess you could do a lot worse than this kindly looking and safely dead Australian who so impressed some of the most penetrating thinkers of the Twentieth Century.

ALTERNATIVE HEALTH NEWS ONLINE

http://altmedicine.com/

This is an outstanding site, created and maintained
by journalist and retired professor Frank Grazian.
It offers sensible, well-written, well-organized news
and opinions about many aspects of alternative medicine.

Yes, it's got it all: great organization, snazzy graphics, carefully attributed articles, and popular style married to serious scholarship. No wonder it was named a "Best of Health & Medicine on the Web" site by NetGuide magazine.

It is gratifying to see that it has been rewarded with great popularity. Frank reports a total of 158,719 hits in three months. Although there is a small amount of advertising at the site, it is clearly marked as such, relatively unobtrusive, and certainly does not appear to affect editorial content.

The "Health News Bulletins," written by Frank himself, are a treasure. He has searched the best of both conventional and unconventional sources to cull the most provocative news items about the benefits—and sometimes the risks—of natural treatments.

Emphasis here is on vitamins and minerals, with short articles such as "Vitamin D is Vital to Good Health." Frank reads widely, loves his subject, and it shows.

Other topics:

Antioxidant Levels and Heart Disease: They report on a study conducted in Sweden which discovered that high mortality from heart disease may be related to low levels of antioxidants. Surprise, surprise. But the Abstract is right there, to check the science for yourself and to print out for your doctor's continuing education.

Frank also reports on a letter in the New England Journal of Medicine—which had gotten past me—on how aspirin and the popular herb ginkgo may not mix well and may in fact cause unwanted bleeding. Although there is a minimum of editorializing here, Frank does quietly point out that bioflavonoids might be used to prevent this from happening—a solution the NEJM letter writers apparently did not consider.

To give an idea of the richness of this site, let us consider just the section on Mind-Body medicine. After an overview on "the latest leading-edge therapies that show how the mind exerts a significant impact on the body," there are descriptions, articles and links to the following approaches:

Art Therapy • Music Therapy • Self-Help Psychology • Hypnosis • Progressive Relaxation • Relaxation Response • Transcendental Meditation • Yoga Paths • Prayer Therapy • Humor Therapy • Guided Imagery • Biofeedback • Meditation and Relaxation • Zen Meditation

What's great about this site is that it provides a handrail for your tour of some very strange areas. To switch metaphors, it projects the enjoyable tension of the borderland between two very different cultures, where the seemingly contradictory collide and occasionally merge in unexpected ways.

You will find alternative practices here cheek-by-jowl with standard science. Frank himself blends traditional, pencil-behind-the-ear journalism with the wild abandon of Internet "e-zines;" In other words, he tempers wide-eyed wonder with a healthy dose of skepticism.

ALTERNATIVE MEDICINE DIGEST

http://www.alternativemedicine.com/

This is another very valuable alt.med. site on the Internet. It is the Cyberspace version of a surprisingly slick magazine, called Alternative Medicine Digest, which promises to make the whole topic of holistic health very accessible to the masses.

The Digest, and matching Web site, is a branch of the Burton Goldberg publishing empire. Mr. Goldberg is a retired business-man with an enormous enthusiasm for his topic. And he has the means to make his dream happen. He wants to be popular, and features movie stars on his covers. Yet he has not sold out to commercial interests and is not afraid to take on some powerful figures in the medical establishment, such as the commissioner of the FDA. His magazine's tone remains militant, indignant and combative.

It will therefore not please everyone, including some of those on the academic side of alternative medicine. Nevertheless, there is a great deal of value here. The site contains the current issue of the Digest. Articles focus on such things as natural remedies for migraine headaches, weight loss success stories, and the feature interview with some celebrity. The month I reviewed the site the beneficiary of this star treatment was singer and talk show host John Tesh. (We learn that John keeps himself healthy with chiropractic, diet, massage, and supplements).

The same issue contained a detailed article about a Mexican cancer clinic with which I am quite familiar. While the coverage was pretty accurate, as accurate as popular journalism generally gets, the tone was highly propagandistic. I agreed with the author's basic point of view, so I should have been pleased. But there were no nuances, shadows, or second thoughts. So it read a bit like a puff piece. A skeptic might dismiss this piece as bought-and-paid-for journalism. But the magazine isn't written for skeptics.

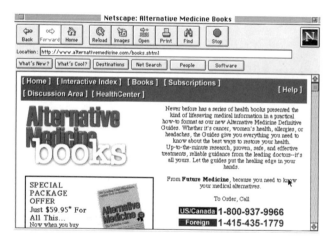

There is also quite a bit of braggadocio at the site. They call themselves the "one-stop read for what's new and effective in alternative medicine." Ugh. The magazine is "The Voice of Alternative Medicine." About their own books, they write, "Never before has a series of health books presented the kind of lifesaving medical information...Whether it's cancer, women's health, allergies, or headaches, the Guides give you everything you need to know...."

I don't think so, but most of the articles in the Alternative Medicine Digest are really pretty good, for they not only summarize important findings and developments in the field but clearly give the medical journal sources of them. Overall, I think they are fulfilling a very useful function. There are pieces that you should have no hesitation in sharing with your doctor, holistic or otherwise.

In summary, my reservations are relatively minor. This is a content-rich site that will come as an eye opener to many people who are unfamiliar with alternative treatments and the growing movement surrounding their use.

ALTERNATIVE MEDICINE CONNECTION

http://www.arxc.com/

In the early '90s, Arline Brecher came to an
Office of Alternative Medicine (OAM) meeting and announced
that she, her husband, and Dr. Charles Farr were planning
an alternative medicine connection on the Internet.
People stared at them blankly. What's the Internet? they asked.

They were true to their word and this was among the first sites concerned with alternative medicine to actually get up and running.

The Alternative Medicine Connection site consists of several discrete parts. First of all, the page that I use almost daily is the trademarked MedSearch. This is a search and referral service for alternative doctors around the US. If you are looking for chelation in Key Largo or a High Colonic in the High Sierras, this is definitely the first place to go.

Here's what they say about themselves:

"Welcome to MedSearch™—the world's most complete directory of holistic practitioners. Although the electronic Yellow Pages includes more than 10,000 health care providers, it is far from complete. Chances are it will never be finished as every day, many more clinicians begin offering holistic health care in response to ever-growing public demand for non-toxic, natural, health-boosting medical care. As this project expands and develops, MedSurfers™ will find here a wealth of information not easily available elsewhere. Those health care providers who choose to do so have the opportunity to tell a great deal about themselves, their specialties, their office practices, their staffing, their education, training, and personal background—as much as they care to reveal."

This site is much stronger in some departments than in others. Let's say, by way of illustration, that a patient in Ten Sleep, Wyoming (population 311) is looking for an alternative practitioner to design a treatment program for himself.

MedSearch quickly locates eight alternative practitioners of all kinds in the state of Wyoming. There turns out to be a bona fide holistic physician (an MD) in the city of Gillette, which is about an hour's drive from his ranch in Ten Sleep. This might be a good match. He will also discover that there's a naturopath in Laramie, a chiropractor in Douglas, etc. Then he can take his pick.

However, there are some serious gaps here, too. Thus, although "Anthroposophically Extended Medicine" (a kind of homeopathy invented by Rudolph Steiner of Waldorf School fame) is listed as a searchable subspecialty, a search turned up zero practitioners of this interesting method in the entire database. So clearly the program has a way to go before it can pretend to completeness; yet it is an excellent beginning and I am sure it has already helped many people.

In addition, the site contains the "Alternative Medicine Connection," which is described as "The world's first OnLine information service dedicated to the scientific and political interests of the holistic health community...a networking tool for organizations wishing to communicate more quickly, efficiently and less expensively."

At the present time, this contains forums and web sites of several organizations. Each time, you have to log onto the site, which is free but extremely annoying. You then have to remember to log off, or else you are "penalized" by a loss of time online. I'm sure there is some "good" reason for this procedure. I found it so off-putting that I will never go back until they change this stupid rule.

Some of the organizations are:
The Great Lakes College of Clinical Medicine
American Preventive Medical Association
Alternative Medicine Media Professionals

Although a frame has been created for these organizations, there is not much meat here yet. One hopes they will be up and running in the near future.

In any case, MedSearch™ alone is worth the visit.

ALTERNATIVE MEDICINE SOURCES

http://www.pitt.edu/~cbw/altm.html

This is the University of Pittsburgh's "jumpstation" for sources of information on unconventional, unorthodox, unproven, or alternative, complementary, innovative, integrative therapies.

This site was created in September, 1994 (which makes it a veteran in Net terms). It is maintained by a librarian, Charles B. Wessel, of the Falk Library of the Health Sciences, University of Pittsburgh who is working under a contract. Although Mr. Wessel is an enthusiast for the general topic, he never lets it show, much less raises his voice above a whisper. It is a huge site. Its weak point is that it is not frequently changed and hadn't been modified in the two months before we last looked.

The site is basically divided into six sections:

1. OAM, Office of Alternative Medicine, NIH
2. Pennsylvania Resources
3. Internet Resources
4. Bibliographic Databases
5. Mailing Lists and Newsgroups
6. Related Resources

1. The OAM information page. This is an independent OAM Web presentation. It offers information about and/or links to the following OAM "exploratory centers." Each of these provides mission statements, some of which are quite lengthy and detailed. (Also see the OAM page at http://altmed.od.nih.gov).

• Bastyr University AIDS Research Center, Alternative Medicine Research in HIV/AIDS

• The Center for Addiction and Alternative Medicine Research, University of Minnesota Medical School & Hennepin County Medical Center

• The Center for Alternative Medicine Research in Cancer, University of Texas, Houston Health Science Center

• Center for Complementary & Alternative Medicine Research in Asthma, Allergy and Immunology, University of California, Davis

• Center for the Study of Complementary and Alternative Therapies (CSCAT), University of Virginia

• Complementary and Alternative Medicine Program at Stanford University (CAMPS), Stanford University

2. Pennsylvania Resources. This lists four places in Pennsylvania that are useful to people interested in alternative medicine. These are the Pittsburgh Center for Natural Health; Point of Light "celebrating wellness of body, heart and soul," a quarterly magazine that provides articles, directories, classifieds and advertisements to health practitioners and products; the Preventative Medicine Center of Sharon and the Whole Health Resources, which offers holistic health counseling. While I am sure these are all good resources, it is unclear why these four were chosen out of many other options.

3. Internet Resources: A large collection of links, but of very varied quality and perspective. You have "QuackWatch," defined as "your guide to health fraud, quackery, and intelligent decision-making" sandwiched between Planet Wellness and the Reiki page.

4. Bibliographic Databases: Similarly, this section offers four choices that are good in and of themselves. But the reason for the choice seems mysterious. They are: Allied and Alternative Medicine (AMED), which provides coverage of complementary or alternative medicine; Manual, Alternative and Natural Therapy (MANTIS) for coverage not significantly represented in the major biomedical databases (not free); Dr. Felix's Free MEDLINE Page; and NAPRALERT, which contains data on natural products.

5. Mailing Lists and Newsgroups: A useful selection of those discussion groups on the Internet relating to alternative medicine.

6. Other Resources: An unusual selection of about a dozen other links of interest, such as Go Ask Alice, an interactive question and answer health line from Columbia University and Self-Help Psychology Magazine, an online educational forum written by mental health professionals and students.

My feeling about the University of Pittsburgh jumpstation is mixed. It was one of the earliest alt.med. sites out of the box and seemed quite fantastic when it first appeared. Now it seems a bit shopworn, especially when compared to other more dynamic sites. When the OAM finally fields its own site, it will be even less critical. However, it is worth a visit, since it still offers a good starting point for a lot of searches.

AMALGAM FILLINGS

http://www.algonet.se/~leif/AmFAQigr.html

One of the hottest controversies in all of medicine concerns the safety of mercury-containing amalgam fillings.

You may not have heard that there are real dentists out there— albeit a distinct minority—who are convinced that mercury-containing fillings (called amalgam fillings in the trade) can cause a whole host of serious diseases, from allergies to cancer.

The thought is staggering, since there are about 100 million amalgam fillings installed each year in the United States alone. If even a tiny percentage of these result in some form of chronic illness, then over the years millions of people will be made sick by this one "innocuous" procedure.

But do amalgams really cause such illnesses? The short answer is: nobody knows. In 1993, the US Department of Health and Human Services, always a conservative voice in health debates, declared, "The possibility that this material, as well as currently available alternatives, could pose health risks cannot be totally ruled out because of the paucity of definitive human studies."

Now they tell me—after a succession of cheery dentists have

packed this stuff into half the teeth in my mouth!

I like this site for two reasons:

First, I think it addresses a really serious question. I am a bit biased. In the summer of 1990, I had the pleasure of dropping in on a Colorado Springs dentist named Hal Huggins, who is the guru of the whole anti-amalgam crowd. Some of his amalgam-removal patients made a deep impression on me.

A woman with multiple sclerosis was now out of her wheelchair for the first time in years. I heard anecdotes of leukemia patients who had "spontaneous remissions" after they had their teeth yanked for other purposes. Apparently such stories are whispered about by dentists in unguarded moments.

I also must say that since then, I have known some individuals, initially enthusiastic about the procedure, who seemed to get a lot worse after they had their fillings removed. I would like somebody to get to the truth of this matter.

Second, I think this site is a model for how to deal with controversial issues in a fair-minded and dispassionate way. The National Cancer Institute gets $2 billion per year in taxpayer money, and yet their discussion of alternative treatments is a joke: error-filled, grossly biased, filled with special pleading for their own treatments.

This site by contrast is fact-filled, well-organized, objective, detailed, and provides scientific references, both pro AND con.

And the funny thing is, it is the product of a single determined individual, Leif Hedegard of Stockholm, Sweden. To add to the wonder, the site is in English, yet English is clearly not even his native language. The AMA's Dr. Lundberg can scoff at "vanity publishing" on the Net. Yet his organization could learn a thing or two from this middle-of-the-night HTML scripter.

Here's what Leif disarmingly writes about himself:

"I am 37 years old. I have worked 10 years as an army officer, three years with mentally disabled children and currently I am working at a school trying to be a part of a good learning environment around information-technique/computers. For 2.5 years I studied in a medical school, but could not manage to succeed with both that and taking care of my son Johan (now 8 years old). Therefore I decided to end my medical training and am now happy about the good contact I have with my son."

Where but on the Internet do you get to meet such people?

See also: http://www.simwell.com/hda/

The above is the site of the Holistic Dental Association, headquartered in Durango, Colorado. (What is it about Colorado and weirdo dentistry?)

AMRTA

http://www.teleport.com:80/~amrta/overview.html

The Alchemical Medical Research and Teaching Association, a mixture of fascinating alternative and esoteric stuff with hard-core research.

'Alchemical Medical Research' doesn't sound very promising. However, despite the New Age title, this happens to be a scientifically sound site. They also run the Paracelsus listserv. Busy folks.

Unfortunately, the authors and/or Webmasters of the site are not identified by name. Maybe that's the alchemical way, but it makes me uneasy. I like to know whom I'm dealing with.

That said, I do appreciate the scope this site provides. For instance, you can find a great many valuable documents here. There is, picking almost at random, a lecture on "Plant Pharmacy" by John Uri Lloyd (1849-1936), who was a celebrated herbalist and founder of the Lloyd Brothers Pharmacy in Cincinnati. According to the authors, "he was perhaps the only true American alchemist." There they go with that "alchemy" again. Where Lloyd's alchemy comes in, however, we are not told. I'm not sure I want to know.

You may not actually learn at this site how to turn base metals into gold. However, a lot of people will appreciate the detailed and practical tips on how to quit smoking. (It starts by setting a quit date, and ends with the hearty advice to "Keep at it. Quitting is the best thing you are doing to improve your life.")

The section on "Understanding Ourselves" gets into some more esoteric material. Take for example an essay with the provocative title, "The Shadow and Physical Symptoms." I was prepared for diagnosing physical illnesses by analyzing your shadow on the sidewalk. (A great topic for the Learning Annex, by the way.) Instead, the word "shadow" is being used in a religio-psychologico-metaphoric sense:

"The 'shadow'...embodies the sum of all those rejected aspects of reality which people either cannot or will not see within themselves, and of which they are therefore unconscious. The shadow is our greatest threat (and ally), because it is always there even though we do not know it or recognize it. It is the shadow that sees to it that all our efforts and purposes eventually turn into their opposites....In summary: dis-ease is the path of the shadow, of integration."

I don't know what it means, but I do enjoy reading it.

I also liked this section on how "The Body Reveals the Spirit":

"'The body never lies.' Its tensions and movements, tone and color, posture and proportions, all express the person and the vitality within. The body speaks of one's emotional history and deepest feelings, one's personality and character. A drooping head, slumped shoulders, a caved-in chest, and a slow, burdened gait reflect feelings of weakness and defeat; while a head carried erect, shoulders straight and loose, a chest breathing fully and easily, and a light gait tell of energy and confident promise."

Telling a child to stand up tall isn't enough; you have to give the child reason to want to stand up tall. Words of wisdom.

There's much, much more here, including such fascinating topics as:

The Body in Mind • Sabbath of Women • Process Paradigm • Master Gardener (imagery) • Inner Guides (imagery) • Healing Belief Systems • Energy centers—Heart • Converting a Symptom to a Signal • Energy Work for Cardio-thoracic Surgery Patients •

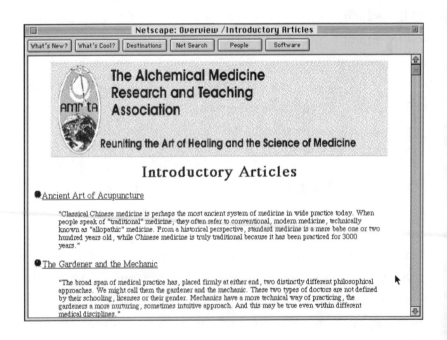

APITHERAPY

http://www.beesting.com/

Make a beeline for BeeOnline,
The Online Publication of the American Apitherapy Society.
It contains a wealth of useful information.

What's New • The Society • How to Get Started • Products From The Hive • Apiary Techniques • Conference Reports • Bee Links

We learn at this site that the use of insects and insect products in medicine began in the distant past. For instance, the use of honey as a medicine is recorded in the Sumerian records of 4,000 BCE (and it's still considered an outstanding dressing for wounds). Something called "bee ointment" was used in Ancient Egypt, and both Pliny and Galen wrote about it. Hippocrates, the patron saint of alternative doctors, said that honey "cleans sores and ulcers of the lips, heals carbuncles and running sores."

Notice the URL, however. What we're mainly talking about here is grabbing bees in a pair of tweezers and applying them to parts of your body, in the hope they will sting you. There is a determined group of people who are sure this is a tremendously effective way to relieve arthritis. Emperor Charlemagne and Ivan the Terrible are said to have used bee stings to relieve joint disease. In fact, the first clinical studies using bee sting for rheumatic disease dates to 1864.

Bee venom therapy had a vogue in the 1930s, but then like most natural treatments went into steep decline. Today, "the majority of classic handbooks on rheumatology...consider it a dubious method, admitting at most its histamine-like and counter-irritant effect."

My guess is—and it is just a guess—that this probably works. I am glad to read that there are now controlled clinical trials underway to scientifically test the alleged benefits of this unusual treatment.

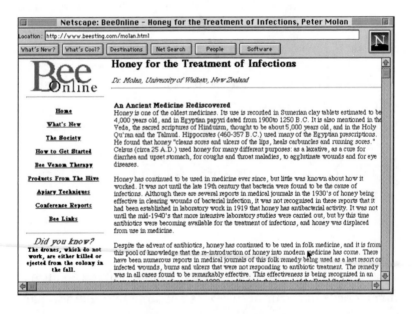

"Formal research in the clinical effects of Bee Venom Therapy (BVT) has just received a significant boost," we are told. "A study on BVT in the treatment of multiple sclerosis, headed by Ross Hauser, MD, was just approved by the Institutional Review Board of the American College for Advancement in Medicine (ACAM, see above). The study is now accepting patients for enrollment."

This is a very rich site, which will sting many people into at least responding to its claims. Bee therapy has many applications, especially but not limited to diseases such as rheumatoid arthritis.

It is potentially a very inexpensive and accessible medicine, which could teach a new respect for beneficial insects around the world. (Of course, since the bee dies after utilizing its sting, it may have a different opinion on the matter.)

ARTHRITIS

http://www.mall-net.com/arth/

A general compendium of forbidden "cures" of arthritis.

According to this site, when your doctor says it can't be cured, s/he generally means that the multi-billion dollar pharmaceutical industry is not interested in finding a cure. "Only YOU can find your own cure for the many diseases called 'Rheumatoid Arthritis," we read. " I hope you check every one of these links. You never know which one will lead You to YOUR cure."

This site links to a great many places where alternative treatments for this painful and disabling condition are to be found. Make sure to take a peek at the "Arthritis Chat" page where individuals counsel each other. This could be most helpful and informative.

"Wilson's Syndrome." According to the literature found here, "If you have a body temperature of less than 98.6° F. and some of the following symptoms you probably have Wilson's Syndrome. This condition involves a disorder where the cells of the body are unable to convert the inactive thyroid hormone, T4, into the more active hormone, T3. Wilson's Syndrome itself does not alter the thyroid hormone tests. It may exist in association with true hypothyroidism, however. In these cases, thyroid tests may be abnormal but the usually prescribed thyroid hormones may not entirely solve the problem."

The symptoms in question include acid indigestion, allergies, anxiety, panic attacks, arthritis, muscular/joint aches, asthma, bad breath, increased bruising, canker sores, carpal tunnel syndrome, elevated cholesterol levels, cold hands and feet and Raynaud's phenomenon, constipation/irritable bowel syndrome, lack of coordination, depression, dry eyes/blurred vision, dry hair, hair loss, dry skin, fatigue, fluid retention, flushing, food cravings, food intolerances, headaches including migraines.

It also cites hemorrhoids, hives, hypoglycemia, recurrent infections, infertility, insomnia and narcolepsy, irregular periods and menstrual cramps, irritability, itchiness, lightheadedness, low blood pressure, decreased memory and concentration, decreased motivation/ambition, musculoskeletal strains, unhealthy nails, changes in pigmentation, skin, and hair, increased post-prandial response, premenstrual syndrome, psoriasis.

Psychological symptoms include: decreased self-esteem, decreased sex drive and anhedonia, inhibited sexual development, increased susceptibility to substance abuse, abnormal swallowing and throat sensations, sweating abnormalities, tinnitus (ringing in the ears), inappropriate weight gain, decreased wound healing.

The trouble with syndromes like this is that most people have half a dozen or more of these symptoms, and many of them also have temperatures below 98.6° F. So apparently most of the population has Wilson's syndrome. This sort of grandiose thinking is what gives alternative medicine a bad name. Nevertheless, as in many things, there could be a kernel of truth here. If you feel it is worth exploring, then this is the site to begin from.

BACH FLOWER REMEDIES

http://www.a-z.co.uk/health/bchquest.htm

I don't know how they work, but many individuals really seem to be helped. Especially valuable is the Rescue Remedy.
Keep this handy for bad news. Even if these are just placebo, the price is low and you are unlikely to do any harm.

Dr. Edward Bach started out as a conventional Harley Street (London) doctor. Midway in his illustrious career, he experienced a kind of religious conversion and fell deeply in love with the flowers and trees he would see on country walks.

He started to prepare extracts of these botanicals and ascribe to them almost mystical properties. Each plant corresponded to a particular mood causing human unhappiness. By taking a microdose of the plant, you corrected these negative emotional states.

I like the Bach remedies. They are inexpensive, self-administered, and highly poetic in a kind of Edwardian way. This site provides the standard Bach flower brochure that you find in health food stores, but in a handy cyber form.

What they say: "The Remedies cover all known negative states of mind from which mankind is known to suffer. They address the imbalance to alter the negative emotional state to a positive one— a positive state of mind will greatly assist in physical recovery and inhibit symptoms from returning."

This site is part of a larger project called the Mystical Crystal. The parent body contains all sorts of esoteric stuff, some of which falls off my personal map. For instance, you can find out about attending what is called an "Atlantean Weekend," where you will learn how "in the older Atlantean civilization, crystals were used quite extensively, and misused to such a degree that they eventually led to the catastrophe which caused Atlantis to disappear into the ocean."

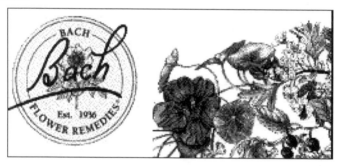

As with everything Atlantean, there is an epistomological puzzle, i.e., how do you get information about a continent that was supposedly destroyed root and branch thousands of years ago? "Our chief sources of information" for the weekend "comes from a number of psychics, who have described for us, each in their own way, yet in strikingly similar depictions, the Atlantean technology of crystal power." Sure.

You will find some amazing stuff here, however. There is, for instance, the International Past-Life Therapists' Directory. These are special people who can allegedly find a link between your current problems and bad stuff that happened to you in your putative past.

Call me a New York skeptic, but I am perpetually amazed at the fact that most people who get regressed in this way find out that they were famous and distinguished individuals in past lives—the Queen of Sheba seems to pop up quite frequently. Few are ever told, "You were a totally insignificant Roman galley slave."

The site also contains:
The International Crystal Healer Directory
The International Yoga Directory
The International Reiki Directory
The International Sound Healer Directory

I have fun thinking about this stuff, and if you don't get too serious about it, you may too.

BASTYR UNIVERSITY

http://www.bastyr.edu/

For those who are interested in the high end of
alternative medicine education, this is an indispensible site.

Bastyr College—now Bastyr University—was founded in 1978 by its eponymous hero, the naturopath John Bastyr. At the time, there wasn't much prestige to being a naturopath. The profession, which had flourished in the early part of the century, was at an all-time low. Yet, look at it now!

In the 1990s, it received the first grant ever to a naturopathic institution by the US government's National Institutes of Health (NIH). This grant created a huge controversy in the New York Times and elsewhere, as critics charged that Bastyr scientists were just too inexperienced to administer such grants, much less perform the work.

Sour grapes. Some allopaths just hated to see any naturopathic institution getting a tiny fraction of the government's largesse, much less the recognition implicit in such funding.

At this well-turned-out site, you can read about the Bastyr University Research Institute, which is conducting 18 separate research projects into natural medicine practices, exploring new treatments for serious chronic diseases, and continuing to develop the faculty's research skills and training students in research methods. They are particularly involved in finding some natural approaches to the AIDS problem, under the leadership of Carlo Calabrese, ND and Leanna Standish, a serious researcher who has both a PhD and ND degrees and used to teach at "establishment" institutions before her "conversion" to naturopathy.

Overall, the emphasis at Bastyr is on combining science with natural medicine. The Web site offers a good overview of this bastion of naturopathy. You will find out about their comprehensive, 1,000-page textbook of naturopathic treatments, which is for sale. (Unfortunately the textbook itself is not online.) You can also find out about Distance Learning— courses for credit that you can take by mail and by computer.

What they say about themselves:

"Bastyr University was founded in 1978 to train naturopathic physicians with a scientific approach. Since then, degree programs in nutrition, acupuncture and Oriental medicine, and applied behavioral science have been added, expanding the mission to serve as an effective leader and a vital force in the improvement of the health and well-being of the human community."

They seem to be fulfilling this mission very effectively.

DR. BOWER

http://galen.med.virginia.edu/~pjb3s/
Complementary_Practices.html

Dr. Peter J. Bower's Complementary and Alternative Medicine
Page — one of the premier Internet resources on alt.med.

This celebrated site is an incredible resource, a mega-jump-station
of Web resources. Under each category is listed dozens, sometimes
hundreds, of other sites dealing with particular topics.

As far as I can see, there is no real attempt made here to winnow
out the wheat berries from the chaff. Consequently, the areas vary
greatly in depth and number. I counted an incredible 468 sites on
acupuncture; on the other hand, there were only 22 sites about
cancer, and about half of those were the NCI/PDQ statements (the
very picture of prejudice). Not surprisingly, a fair number are
"duds" (inactive links). There are also some ridiculous mis-
spellings (Dr. Max Gerson becomes Dr. Gearson).

By and large, however, this super site makes up in sheer quantity
for small technical errors. It is exuberant in its enthusiasm for the
galactic vastness of the Internet. If you have an intense interest in
any particular alternative medical topic, this is as good a jumping
off point as you are likely to find.

BURZYNSKI

http://catalog.com/bri/bri.htm

Not every alternative cancer doc makes it to the front page of the New York Times! Stanislaw Burzynski, MD, PhD, is a Houston physician who, in a celebrated trial, was exonerated of all charges of violating FDA's laws.

Antineoplastons are non-toxic substances that have shown most promising in the treatment of difficult brain cancers and non-Hodgkins lymphoma. At this site you can find out about the Burzynski Research Institute (BRI) and how to start antineoplaston treatment at this Houston, Texas clinic.

You can submit an application electronically. (There are times when it is impossible to get through to BRI by telephone.) Their Informational Brochure is also available online as are a number of other supporting materials.

Against all odds, Dr. Burzynski's combative institute continues to operate, to treat patients and to conduct clinical trials of antineoplastons, which are non-toxic substances that have been reported to produce results in the treatment of various kinds of cancer.

Treatment aside, this Polish-born doctor has taken more arrows than St. Sebastian. A tag team of industries and agencies, prosecutors and persecutors has been trying to put him out of business (and in prison) for almost 20 years. The Aetna Insurance Company, sneering quackbusters, the Texas Board of Medical Examiners, the Food and Drug Administration, the US Justice Department—everyone has gotten a whack at this guy, but he just bounces back. It is an amazing spectacle of perseverance in the face of adversity.

Burzynski, and his Patient Relations Director, Dean Mouscher, were among the first to recognize the role that the Internet could play in shaping public opinion. They put government documents and correspondence up on their site and during his trial provided a blow-by-blow report of the on-going events. I turned to it frequently.

They were quick to point out that Burzynski Research Institute is conducting 68 FDA-approved clinical trials of antineoplastons in the treatment of cancer—while at the same time being prosecuted by the FDA. Patients and concerned citizens were encouraged to call the President and their Congressmen. This Web site therefore exerted a real influence on public policy.

You will find evidence here that as early as 1991 government officials knew and acknowledged that the anticancer effects of antineoplastons were real. Yet they stepped up their prosecution from that point, threatening to pull the rug out from under patients on the treatment. You can also read Burzynski's side as to why the NCI/Sloan-Kettering/Mayo Clinic trials of antineoplastons were really cancelled. This Web site is exciting. A pioneering effort in every way.

BUTEYKO

http://www.gil.com.au/~pathein/video/method.html

If you or someone you know suffers from a
breathing disorder—emphysema, bronchitis, allergy,
sinus infection, and especially asthma—
you definitely will want to check out this site.

The Buteyko site offers information on what is called "ICDR" or
more popularly, the Buteyko Method. According to its passionate
proponents, this "is the most effective known natural method,
which is drug-free and gives quick results for asthmatics of any
severity."

At this site, they do not hesitate to use the word "cure" in connection with the treatment, which has created a great deal of controversy. After practicing this technique for six weeks, they say, asthma sufferers on average reduce their use of inhalers by 90 percent.
That sounds like a cure, for sure.

I cannot judge the validity of this treatment, but the site itself is
straightforward, fact-filled and credible. I got excited reading it,
since I knew nothing whatsoever about this controversy. The site
is maintained by patients, and they say that none is affiliated with
a clinic offering this treatment. Webmaster is Peter Kolb, an
Australian biomedical engineer. The only commercial product

sold on the site is a video tape about Buteyko. They also offer access to a Buteyko mailing list.

This site narrates the fascinating story of Professor Konstantin Buteyko, a Russian physician who discovered in 1953 that deep respiration (which I gather is another name for hyperventilation) can actually be a serious condition. That is because it can serve as a prelude to a number of other secondary diseases, among which is asthma. Since 1980, they say, Buteyko therapy has been the standard treatment for asthma in Russia, although it is little known or recognized in the West.

They reprint a very technical 20-page article by the great Buteyko himself. It is written in turgid European-style scientific prose, and then translated rather awkwardly into English, adding another layer of obscurity. But with all that, I could tell that the man is extremely learned and possibly brilliant.

If one is suffering from any of the above mentioned breathing diseases, it would certainly be worth serious effort to download and study this and related articles. Or you can cut to the bottom line and just try the method itself.

For reasons unknown, however, the method is very popular in the United Kingdom and the Commonwealth countries, such as Australia and New Zealand, but virtually unknown in the US and other places.

One force behind its popularization has been some prominent athletes. The former squash champion Carin Clonda, herself a chronic asthmatic, claims that a course in the Buteyko treatment saved her from a debilitating condition in which medication was having no effect. It is also said that one hundred of Australia's top athletes are currently involved in research testing this method.

What they say: "Chris Drake's sessions at the Hale Clinic in London begin with a 'controlled pause'. Anyone can do it, he says, and it will tell you if you are over-breathing. Breathe in gently for two seconds, out for three seconds, then hold your breath until it becomes uncomfortable. Less than 10 seconds and you have a serious health problem, less than 25 and you are unhealthy, 30 to 40 is OK and 60 plus excellent.

"On the second day, the hard work of improving the controlled pause begins. Participants fight the urge to breathe in and gradually, the time they can manage increases. By the third day, results are starting to appear." (Reprinted from The Independent Newspaper, UK, June 10, 1996.)

For more conventional information about asthma, check out: http://www.radix.net/ ~ mwg/asthma-gen.html

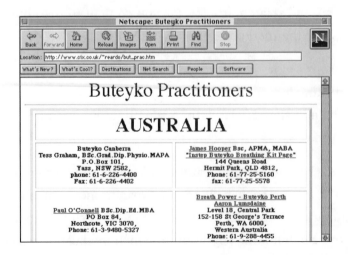

CANCERGUIDE

http://cancerguide.org/

Steve Dunn's Cancer Information Page.
Steve is a long-term survivor of kidney cancer, who created
and maintains this comprehensive site for other patients.

CancerGuide has a wide variety of information, both orthodox and unorthodox, on cancer treatments. Steve is not afraid to give his personal views. A very worthwhile site.

This is another of those remarkable sites that is the product of one determined individual. Steve provides the following classes of information:

Basic Information on Cancer and CancerGuide. Under this, he offers an interesting section on the "pros and cons of researching your cancer." Not everyone is ready to become their own researcher, and Steve recognizes that. He also provides a guide to understanding adjuvant chemotherapy (written by Kevin Murphy, MD) and another on "understanding pathology reports." There is the provocative "fear and loathing in the ICU" and a guide to "thinking rationally about side effects." Hot topics, all.

He offers fellow patients advice on what to do if they have a rare cancer or if they are confronting the prospect of a bone marrow transplant.

And what about alternative treatments?

Well, Steve has two sections, one on "unconventional" approaches, the other on alternatives. What he calls "unconventional" approaches are new ideas about conventional treatment, such as chemosensitivity testing or conservative surgery. He also offers a dozen articles about some of the more prominent alternative treatments. Thus:

Some Thoughts on Evaluating Alternative Therapies

Recommended Books on Alternative Therapies

PSK: A Non-Toxic Anti-Tumor Polysaccharide

Bovine Cartilage

Charles B. Simone's Shark Cartilage Protocol

Antineoplastons/Burzynski Clinic

Coley's Toxins/Fever Therapy

Gerson Therapy

Sun Soup

Elixir Vitae

Information on Essiac

Info on Gaston Naessens' 714-X

Hulda Clark's "The Cure for All Cancers"

His approach is open-minded yet adequately skeptical, a useful mindset for patients entering this slippery field. Steve himself is disarming in his honesty. For example, about the Hulda Clark anti-parasite "cure for all cancers," he writes:

"I'm going to admit to you right up front that I haven't carefully researched Hulda Clark's theories. In fact, I've spent a total of about fifteen minutes looking over her book, The Cure For All Cancers, in a local health food store. That's all the time I needed to figure out if there is anything worthwhile there....

"When I looked at The Cure for All Cancers, the first thing that caught my eye was the list of 100 documented cases. To paraphrase the watchwords of the '92 Clinton Campaign, "It's the Data, Stupid!" So I turned right to the cases to see what there was, and what I saw," says Dunn, "was 'Stupid Data'.... Hulda Clark's cases are classic examples of rotten methodology."

It's not politically correct, to be sure, and he's bound to p.o. some true believers, but he's telling you how it looks to someone who's really been there...and back.

I list this site first among all the links I provide at my own Cancer Chronicles site. Simply put, it's a gem.

CANCER CHRONICLES

http://www.ralphmoss.com

A comprehensive collection of articles
on alternative and complementary treatments for cancer,
together with a hard hitting critique of the failure
of the war on cancer.

I blush. This is my own site, my own baby. How can I be objective about something I have spent so many hours crafting? I can't, but I'll describe it for you, briefly, and hope you will go there and make up your own mind.

There is a wealth of information at this site for the person concerned with cancer and its treatments. The Cancer Chronicles, which is now online here, continues the tradition of a printed newsletter by that name, which was available by subscription only from 1989 through the beginning of 1997. Now we have stopped print publication and thrown in our lot entirely with the Internet.

Since we offer this information for free, we have lost the income we derived from the newsletter. On the other hand, whereas we struggled in the past to find readers who wanted and needed this sort of information, we are currently attracting thousands of visitors per month to the site. At the rate we are going, I imagine that we will soon be seeing 100,000 hits before long. Given the fairly esoteric nature of the subject, I do not imagine The Chronicles would have attracted that kind of audience in a print medium.

In addition, I am thrilled by the international nature of the crowd that is coming to visit us every day. Alternative medicine is all about internationalism. Here is a list of the countries whose residents have come to our Web site in one four-month period, given in the order of frequency of their visits:

USA	New	Denmark	Slovenia	Portugal	Estonia
Canada	Zealand	Singapore	Romania	Indonesia	Malta
Australia	Japan	Israel	Taiwan	Philippines	Croatia
United	Belgium	Thailand	Poland	Ireland	Bermuda.
Kingdom	Brazil	Sweden	Switzerland	Brunei	
Spain	France	Austria	Egypt	Trinidad	
Malaysia	Germany	Netherlands	Anguilla	and Tobago	
Russia	Italy	South Africa	Chile	Bahamas	
Norway	Colombia	Greece	Venezuela	Mexico	

One of the first things we did was to upload over 200 articles from back issues of The Cancer Chronicles to the site. (One woman recently informed me that she had downloaded 150 separate items in one busy day.) These are sub-divided into ten separate categories and cover a wide variety of topics, medical and political.

I believe that this constitutes a comprehensive archive of information about non-toxic cancer treatments and the on-going struggle to defend freedom of choice in medicine. It is provided as a public service to patients and to all those who are interested in the development of more effective and humane ways of approaching the cancer problem. I often worried about the fate of all those articles in my personal archives. So for me as an author there is something wonderful about knowing that my work—which would otherwise be gathering dust on the shelf—is out in the world, having an effect. The Internet as Immortality.

When the decision to abandon the printed newsletter was made, some wondered if there really would be a online version. After all, the newsletter was now provided for free, and no one was owed anything. It has surprised me how eager we are to get news to the online community. It has revitalized the effort. Each issue shapes up and is added to continually. To give you some idea of what we're doing, a recent issue contains the following:

The Burzynski Trial. The judge threw out all the fraud charges. Two juries exonerated him. So why does the government pursue an ugly vendetta against this promising treatment?

Oncologist Finds Antineoplastons "Astounding". A Seattle oncologist has declared Burzynski's results in brain cancer "astounding." But will Judge Lake listen?

Deadly Medicine. A review of a book on the deaths of tens of thousands of people from taking FDA approved medications.

Dr. Max. A review of a new biographical novel about the life and works of Dr. Max Gerson, founder of a school of diet therapy.

Selenium and Dr. Revici. How we may be able to prevent about half of all cancers.

Return of The Grape Cure. Science discovers benefits of an old "cure."

Philly's Paper Has Got Right Attitude. Restoring common sense to the medical debate.

The Conversion of Ms. Jane Brody. Even the New York Times registers some changes.

Dangers of Hormone Replacement. How safe is this popular mixture?

At our site we also offer brochures and information on our Healing Choices cancer consultation service, and about our Equinox Press books and tapes. These include The Cancer Industry, Cancer Therapy and Questioning Chemotherapy, as well as Anne Beattie's See Yourself Well relaxation and visualization tapes. In fact, whatever we're doing is likely to find its way onto the Web site.

For me personally, the Internet has put some of the excitement back into writing. From a writer's point of view, who could ask for anything more?

CHANTILLY REPORT

http://199.170.0.141/uctreport/toc.htm

This is one of the best things the US government
has published on complementary medicine.
It is called "Alternative Medicine: Expanding Medical Horizons,"
but is more popularly known as the "Chantilly Report."

The Chantilly Report was prepared under the auspices of the National Institutes of Health's memorable Workshop on Alternative Medicine, held September 14-16, 1992. The Report itself was published by the Government Printing Office.

Working on this report, and relating to the "extended family" that produced it, occupied much of my time and energy for years. As with the previous site it is difficult for me to write about this dispassionately. As I look over the online version I am afflicted by waves of nostalgia for that high tide of enthusiasm we felt as we worked on this effort.

The brief history is this. The Office of Alternative Medicine (OAM) was established in 1991, with the appropriation of a measly $2 million from the US Congress for the creation of an office to "more adequately explore unconventional medical practices."

Senator Tom Harkin's (D-IA) Senate Appropriations Committee had acknowledged that "many routine and effective medical procedures now considered commonplace were once considered unconventional and counterindicated." Cancer radiation therapy was given as an example of "a procedure that is now commonplace but once was considered to be quackery."

The first public meeting to explore the scope of the new office was held in Bethesda, Maryland on June 17-18, 1992. (Several speeches to that meeting are posted to The Cancer Chronicles site.) Under the guidance of Dr. Steven Groft and Dr. Jay Moskowitz, soon to become Acting Director of NIH, a huge meeting of experts was convened three months later.

This was to be one of the seminal events in the history of alternative medicine in the United States. Since the event was held at a posh resort in Chantilly, Virginia, it has come to be known as the Chantilly meeting.

A total of more than 200 participants discussed the state of the art in all the identifiable major areas of alternative medicine. We directed our collective attention to what we considered the "priority areas for potential future research activities."

At Steve Groft's urgent request, the cochairs of the Workshop's working groups organized writing teams to collect and synthesize the available research in their respective fields and to develop recommendations to the National Institutes of Health (NIH) on what research needed to be done in this field. The goal was a big book that could serve as a state-of-the-art report.

The Editorial Board was chaired by Brian Berman, MD and David

Larson, MD. Between 1992 and 1995, we spent hundreds of hours writing, editing and debating the minutiae of the report. Finally, against all odds, it was published by the Government Printing Office, the first time in history that the United States government had issued such a serious (and generally sympathetic) investigation of this field.

But everything that happened around this report afterwards was a big letdown. NIH simply did not disseminate or publicize it in a serious way. It has had very limited distribution, which is a pity. That is why I was thrilled to see it brought back to life on the Net. It is significant that at the moment it is being disseminated online not by the NIH itself but by a group of determined alt.med. activists (affiliated with the "Natural Health Village").

My only criticism of the online version is that it is in tiny type. Serious readers would be well advised to spare their precious eyesight and print it out in a comfortable-to-read version.

Here are the contents, which should give an idea of the phenomenal scope of this historic project. You should know that the report contains hundreds, possibly thousands, of references for further study, most of them from peer-reviewed studies. Not all of these are online.

Part I: Fields of Practice
Mind-Body Interventions
Bioelectromagnetic Applications in Medicine
Alternative Systems of Medical Practice
Manual Healing Methods
Pharmacological and Biological Treatments

Herbal Medicine

Diet and Nutrition in the Prevention and Treatment of
  Chronic Disease

Part II: Conducting and Disseminating Research
Introduction
Research Infrastructure: Institutions and Investigators
Research Databases
Research Methodologies
Peer Review
Public Information Activities

Part III: Conclusion, Appendixes, Glossary, and Index
Conclusion

Also see The OTA Report:
http://199.170.0.141/uctreport/

The same site gives access to another government report, the OTA
Report on Unconventional Cancer Treatments. This was created
by the Office of Technology Assessment between 1986 and 1990.
In retrospect, the OTA project was a way station towards the creation of the Office of Alternative Medicine. I have analyzed
the significance of the OTA Report very extensively at www.
ralphmoss.com.

CHINESE MEDICINE

http://www.rscom.com/tcm/index.html

The Foundation for Traditional Chinese Medicine
and the British Acupuncture Council
run this simple but attractive page.

In 1995, five British organizations concerned with Oriental medicine came together as the British Acupuncture Council (BAcC). I have always believed that the maturation of a field comes about when it starts to discipline (or "police") its own members, winnowing out those practices which can truly be called fraudulent.

Thus, it is auspicious that the BAcC reports that "in addition to governing its members, [it] works to maintain common standards of education, ethics, discipline and Codes of Practice to ensure the health and safety of the public at all times." The BAcC also promotes research and enhances the role that traditional acupuncture can play in the health and well-being of the nation," the nation in question being of course Great Britain.

What conditions can acupuncture treat? According to the World Health Organization (which is turning into a fast friend of alternative medicine), these include a vast panoply:

Upper Respiratory tract	Disorders of the Mouth
Acute sinusitis	Toothache
Acute rhinitis	Post-extraction pain
Common Cold	Gingivitis
Acute tonsilitis	Acute and chronic pharyngitis
Respiratory system	Acute bronchitis
Bronchial asthma	Gastrointestinal system
Spasms of esophagus and cardia	Hiccough
Acute and chronic gastritis	Gastric hyperacidity
Chronic duodenal ulcer (pain relief)	
Acute duodenal ulcer (without complications)	
Acute bacillary dysentery	Constipation
Diarrhoea	Paralytic ileus
Disorders of the Eye	Acute conjunctivitis
Central retinitis	Myopia (in children)
Cataract (without complications)	Neurological and musculoskeletal disorders
Headache	Nocturnal enuresis
Migraine	Intercostal neuralgia
Trigeminal neuralgia	Cervicobrachial syndrome
Facial palsy (early stage)	'Frozen shoulder'
Pareses following a stroke	'Tennis elbow'
Peripheral neuropathies	Sciatica
Sequelae of poliomyelitis (early)	Low back pain
Meniere's disease	Osteoarthritis
Neurogenic bladder dysfunction	

Source: Bannerman R H 1979 Acupuncture: the WHO View. World Health, December, p27-28.

A similar resource for Australia:

http://www2.eis.net.au/ ~ aaca/ Also see:

http://www.qi-journal.com/AcuPoints/acupuncture.html which has an amusing interactive model of the human body with many acupuncture sites. A good use of the online environment.

CHINESE MEDICINE JOURNAL

http://www.pavilion.co.uk/jcm/welcome.html

Web sites on traditional Chinese medicine tend to be poorly written, overly commercial and/or disorganized. This one is different.

This is the online presence of a scholarly journal that was founded in 1979, at a time when information on acupuncture and traditional Chinese medicine was hard to come by.

From the start, its philosophy has been to present "clear, detailed information on basic Chinese medicine theory to a level unavailable elsewhere in English." Since then, they have become recognized as one of the leading journals of all aspects of TCM published in English.

Understandably, this journal is trying to sell subscriptions, and so at this site you will find only a few samples of full-length articles. However, the news section is rather awesome. It contains dozens of short but fascinating news articles on the march of progress of Chinese (and alternative) medicine around the world.

They also present a good Practitioner Reference Guide with an invaluable listing of acupuncture practitioners in the United States.

What I particularly like about this site is that they are not trying to cover up potential problems or difficulties involved in the use of Chinese medicines. Thus, they provide a link to three really excellent articles by Subhuti Dharmananda, PhD, one of the world's leading Oriental medicine researchers who writes about such thorny issues as:

• How Clean and Pure are Chinese Herbs?

• Drugs In Imported Chinese Herb Products; and

• Liver Inflammation Induced By Herbs

These are found at:

http://www.europa.com/ ~ itm/liver.htm
the Institute for Traditional Medicine in Portland, Oregon.

All in all, this, and its linked "friends," provide a superior group of honest and informative sites.

CHIROPRACTIC

http://www.chiro.org/

Chiropractic is one of the original forms of alternative medicine. Chiropractors have been so successful that it is not even clear if they should be called "alternative" anymore.

Chiropractors have survived serious persecution by the AMA. They have gained international approval as a good treatment for lower-back-pain. There are many Web sites concerned with this profession. But many seem unsure of how to relate to their wild past, when the founder, Iowa's Dr. Palmer, walked the earth and challenged the medical profession for control of turf.

Palmer's claims were overstated and hard to justify in the light of science, but in those days chiropractic was an exciting profession that seemed to provide answers. Many chiropractors, judging from their Web sites, are suffering from an identity crisis.

This particular site is not exactly exciting, but is at least lively and youthful. Although oriented towards the professional (while hinting at various splits and divisions) it offers quite a bit of information and even the means of getting a referral to a local practitioner, if that is what you are looking for. This could be helpful for a variety of conditions.

There are interesting historical tidbits here. I also found an abstract on "The Political History of Quackery in Early Century Medical Practice...in Australia, 1870-1914." I always like to curl up with a good history of quackery. But they're so hard to find.

Also see: http://www.chiroweb.com/

This is an an Internet based communications network devoted exclusively to providing information on and for Chiropractors. CHIROWEB provides a way to find a chiropractor almost anywhere in the world. You can enter in information by city and state, by zip or area code. It is admirably complete.

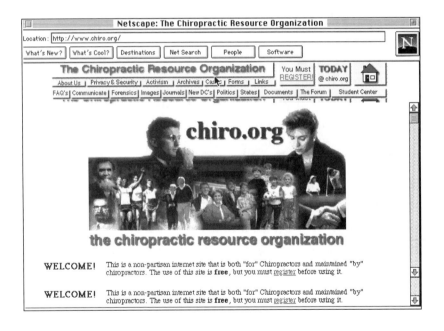

DEEPAK CHOPRA

http://www.randomhouse.com/chopra/

Deepak Chopra is an international "phenom."
His astonishing success—with five bestsellers—
is both cause and effect of
public interest in alternative medicine.

Deepak Chopra has sold over one million copies of "Ageless Body, Timeless Mind" alone. He runs a medical center, gives seminars just about every week, is everywhere on television, and even writes novels and inspirational works about Merlin the Magician. It's as if there were a legion of Chopras, not one mere individual.

Dr. Chopra has engendered his share of controversy and opposition, as well. However, he is clearly a man of extraordinary powers who deserves his success and wears it gracefully. I remember how one afternoon, in 1986, I casually turned on the radio and was absolutely mesmerized by a man with an Indian accent whose words seemed the most brilliant I had heard in years. Uncharacteristically, I turned the apartment upside down until I found a blank tape, threw it in the cassette deck, and then recorded his words. The speaker was Deepak Chopra, before he had gained his current mass appeal.

I am sad to report that this site is not particularly exciting. That may be because it is maintained by his mainstream publisher, Random House. It is clean and neat, but with little actual content. The most interesting thing is the Forum, where people can get to write to Deepak. The Forum seems to make his publisher slightly nervous, for they add a note: "Random House does not necessarily endorse, support, sanction, encourage, verify, or agree with the comments, opinions, or statements posted in the Forum." It is a far cry from Andrew Weil's dynamic "Ask Dr. Weil" website.

The day I looked there were about a dozen new messages from around the world. People write to the doctor with their problems, economic and otherwise. One individual wrote, "I am a thinker. Thinking is what I do. Occasionally...I speak . . . out of context."

No answers were printed online and I could only wonder how the busy Chopra dealt with the outpouring of adulation and human need that comes his way every day.

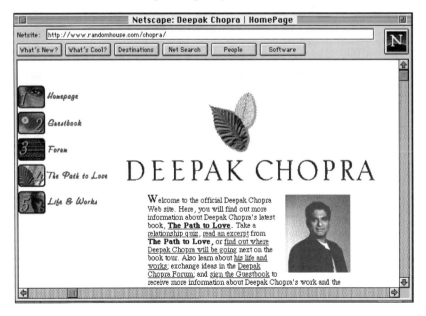

CYBERBOTANICA

http://biotech.chem.indiana.edu/botany/

A knowledge of herbs and their properties is a big part of
alternative medicine. If you slept through botany
here is your chance to redeem yourself,
to master one of the most beautiful of all sciences.

Cyberbotanica is a real find, an exceptionally attractive botany
education resource, maintained by faculty members of Indiana
University. Cyberbotanica will help you get a free online botany
education. It is produced by Lucy Snyder of Indiana University's
BioTech Project.

Eventually they say it will contain chapters on plants used in
bioremediation, on fungi which produce antibiotics, and on genet-
ically engineered fruits and vegetables.

One of the particular interests of this site happens to be botanical
compounds that are used in cancer treatment and research. There
are many. Some of these are non-toxic and therefore (by my definition) fall within the realm of alternative medicine. Others, like
taxol and vincristine, are highly, highly toxic.

There are lovely illustrations and extended descriptions of about
10 such plants (including the Pacific Yew, source of taxol) along
with a table describing more than 60 others. The authors note that

this is not a self-help site. In other words, don't cuddle up with a cup of taxol tea.

The site contains many other interesting and useful sections:

BioTech's Science Dictionary: There are 4,800+ completely searchable dictionary entries on biochemistry, genetics, botany, ecology and more. Bookmark this one if you have a serious interest in the life sciences.

BioTech's Science Resources: Researchers will find resources here on a wide variety of science and biotechnology disciplines as well as explanations of what they are and instructions on how to use them.

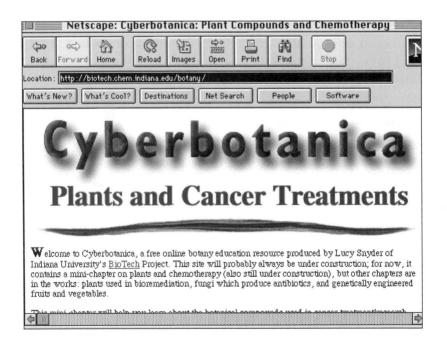

BioTech's Educational Guides: These staff-written guides introduce a wide variety of biotechnology topics, such as proteins, nucleic acids and genetics.

Biotechnology Resource Database / Site Search: You can use it to look up links to other sites based on keywords, or launch an Excite-based search to look for BioTech pages which discuss particular topics.

Professional Resources: Useful for anyone who is considering graduate school, or who is searching for biotechnology researchers, organizations, conferences, or information on biotechnology regulations, commercial vendors, and jobs.

Literature Resources: One can surf through online literature databases and stay up to date on new biotechnology advancements and discoveries with their annotated list of the best science journals and papers on the Web.

A charming and well organized effort from some people who are very serious about their plants.

EMDR

http://www.emdr.com

EMDR—not just a treatment but a movement, which is used to treat problems ranging from trauma to low self-esteem.

Advocates of "Eye Movement Desensitizing and Reprocessing" or EMDR have been attacked by vigilant quackbusters who claim that the method is nothing but a conjuring trick:

"The therapist waves a stick in front of the patient and the patient is supposed to follow the moving stick with his or her eyes" is what they say.

EMDR is interesting. It approaches a number of medical problems handled less than adequately by orthodox medicine. The site itself however is simple, clear-cut, slightly boring. It describes itself as "an interactional, standardized approach and method to therapy that integrates into, and augments, a treatment plan." What prose! "EMDR accelerates the treatment of a wide range of pathologies and self esteem issues related to both upsetting past events and present life conditions.

"Controlled studies of victims of Vietnam combat, rape, molestation, accident, catastrophic loss and natural disaster indicate that the method is capable of a rapid desensitization of traumatic memories, including a cognitive restructuring and a significant reduction of client symptoms (e.g., emotional distress, intrusive thoughts, flashbacks and nightmares."

Advocates claim that there are more controlled studies to date on EMDR than on any other method used in the treatment of trauma. I have no reason to doubt them.

EMDR was developed in 1987 by Francine Shapiro, PhD who is a Senior Research Fellow at the Mental Research Institute, Palo Alto, California. Dr. Shapiro is the recipient of the 1994 Distinguished Scientific Achievement in Psychology Award presented by the California Psychological Association. She is said to have trained over 14,000 clinicians internationally and has used the method in thousands of treatment sessions with patients who had a considerable range of presenting complaints, including having suffered: **rape, sexual molestation, Vietnam combat, natural disaster.**

To date, over 20,000 licensed mental health therapists in 38 countries have been trained in EMDR. Because a clinical background is necessary for the effective application of EMDR, their workshops are limited to mental health professionals who are licensed or certified to provide treatment. Training is considered mandatory for appropriate use. EMDR is a specialized approach and method that requires supervised training for full therapeutic effectiveness and client safety. Clients are at risk if untrained clinicians attempt to use EMDR.

What others say about them:

"EMDR is a powerful tool in the hands of a skillful therapist..I've found it extremely useful in the treatment of the painful aftermath of rape, assault, combat, drug addiction, and the death of a loved one. But I've also found it a real help in overcoming the wide variety of less dramatic issues that bring people into my office: Overcoming jealousy, envy, and the loss of relationships (including divorce), fear of taking a test or fear of an intimidating boss, writer's and artist's block, sexual inhibition, and a variety of self-sabotage."—Lewis Engel, PhD, clinical psychologist, private practice, San Francisco

The most popular book on this topic is EMDR: The Breakthrough Therapy For Overcoming Anxiety, Stress, And Trauma by Francine Shapiro, PhD & Margot Silk Forrest, published by Basic Books, Inc.

RICHARD EVANS, MD

http://web-hou.iapc.net/~raevans/

**Dr. Evans is an experienced Houston surgeon
who devotes himself to promoting rationality
in the field of cancer treatment.**

He represents a conservative philosophy that is quite radical in this day and age. He believes that in many cases "less is more," and that it is not always necessary or desirable for patients to undergo radical surgery or other highly invasive procedures.

His book, Making the Right Choice: Treatment Options in Cancer Surgery, got me so excited that I flew down to Houston to meet the man! I now include this among the "crucial" sites at www.ralphmoss.com. I consult it, and Dr. Evans himself, frequently.

In some ways, this may seem like an odd choice for a book about alternative medicine. Dr. Evans is a Diplomate of the American Board of Surgery and his book was hailed by the thoroughly orthodox American Journal of Surgery in these terms: "This book is excellent. (It) challenges ...surgical tenets that were once etched in stone."

In fact, the book review editor of the Journal of the National Cancer Institute wrote, "Most of the young oncologists I know support Dr. Evans' ideas and have since 1985. Many surgeons are still defending obsolete ideas."

Dr. Evans' logical idea could revolutionize the whole practice of oncology. What he is saying is that radical surgery is essentially unproven, and unjustified in many cases. This is well established now in the case of breast cancer. But he says that there is no proof for the value of radical cutting in most other kinds of cancer as well. Dr. Evans believes in the value of conservative surgery as the treatment of choice for many instances. In other cases, of course, it is necessary to use more radical measures, but each case must be evaluated on an individual basis.

Having met the man, I know that he has put his whole life into preaching this gospel of conservative surgery to both his colleagues and to the general public. He gave up a thriving practice of surgery in order to promote the message of the book.

Is it alternative medicine? I guess that depends on your definition of the field. Alternative medicine is sometimes defined as that which is not taught in medical schools. In that case, it is certainly alternative, since surgeons are still being taught to perform radical surgery in many cases for which, as Evans shows, the data simply do not support such usage.

This is a good example of how alternative medicine can easily make common cause with many of the most embattled figures in conventional medicine, thereby shifting the boundary lines of the struggle.

I myself consider anything that is non-toxic or considerably less toxic than prevailing treatments to be "alternative medicine." I also am drawn to anyone in the healing arts who is unfairly scorned or opposed by his or her colleagues. Thus, although Evans has gotten some support from wise minds in the field, the profession as a whole has gone blithely on its way, unaware that the ground has been cut out from under it.

However, if you are facing cancer surgery I would strongly urge you to at least visit this site, tell your doctor about it, and if warranted, seek out a consultation with Dr. Evans himself. (Information on how to reach him is included at the Web site.) Evans suggests that patients seek out second opinions with those who have opposing views to the doctor giving the first opinion.

In his own words:

"Leading surgeons and scientists have made important new discoveries about the treatment of cancer. They have concluded that most early cancers can be successfully treated with conservative or limited surgery that preserves bodily function and form.

"Careful, scientific studies have proven that cancer cells which may remain following conservative surgery do not spread to other parts of the body. This is one reason conservative surgery is so successful. Surgeons do not have to remove every last cancer cell in one extensive operation. They have a second chance to cure the patient, if the cancer reappears."

(For a reasoned critique of Evans's position see Steve Dunn's CancerGuide, http://cancerguide.org/)

GEMSTONES

http://www.visi.com/~talon/pagan/gems.html

No book about alternative medicine would be complete
without crystals and gemstones. This is the first thing
some people think of when they think of this topic.

I have no idea if gems and minerals really exert a biological effect.
But they can be a lot of fun, as long as an obsession with them
does not become a substitute for more proven medications. If you
are suffering from a serious condition, I think you should check
the results of your gemwork with more objective tests.

I don't know who created this site. The author writes:

"I've created this page using some charts that I've had
laying around as well as from email, web sites, and
other books I've read."

Not a very auspicious start. This site is part of a larger one devoted to magic and paganism. I am sure this will freak out some religious readers, who will see proof of deviltry in it. Personally, one
of the things I like about the Web is that I can encounter the ideas
of people like these anonymous sorcerers without having to
encounter the sorcerers themselves. (I'm assuming their computers are too unsophisticated to trace me back to my home office.)

Anyway, this anonymous site is as good an introduction as you're likely to get to the subject of crystals and gemstones. After an introduction to the elements (fire, air, earth, water and spirit, in case you had forgotten your medieval chemistry), there follows a detailed explanation of the spiritual properties of gems—more gems than you could imagine even exist.

So if you yearn to get started in "crystal work," as they call it, this site has a sensible suggestion: "a quartz crystal with cloudlike 'flaws' is a great (and inexpensive) start. Quartz pebbles are common in pea gravel roads and playgrounds, too, so you can start with that for free." If you ever see me walking country roads, staring deep into the pea gravel, you'll know what I'm doing.

What can I say—I like this site. I like their parsimony. One of the things that has always made me a bit suspicious of gemwork is that it can become a very expensive hobby, very quickly—all for medical claims that have little basis in any science that postdates the Fifteenth Century.

Here you can learn that alexandrite is excellent for "tissue regeneration," especially of the central nervous system. Or that something they call larimar "cools, draws out inflammation, fevers, sunburn heat." Rhodochrosite has "specialized uses to detox/heal blood, liver, cancer." While pink tourmaline is also said to be good for "self-gentleness, especially with severe illnesses like cancer."

There are useful cautionary notes as well: "Be aware—obsidian balls help to see truths by initially amplifying beliefs, patterns, fears, blocking our growth." I'll try to remember that the next time I play with a set of obsidian balls.

Another interesting gem related site is

:http://www.gems4friends.com/ ~lorraine/therapy.html#cln

This is a commercial site reporting the personal opinions of the company's owner, Loretta Elaine. She does not make global statements about the value of gems and crystals but simply tries to provide some high-quality gems and tells you what they seem to have done for her, her family and friends. She seems pretty honest.

Loretta's gems are essentially jewelry (why was I surprised?). They look to me like ordinary earrings and necklaces, pretty nice ones, in fact. However, according to Loretta, wearing such gems actually conveys some subtle influence on one's health and well-being. Loretta tells you about (and can sell you):

Gemstones that encourage change • Gemstones which open the heart • Gemstones for the mind • Gemstones to bring you what you need

There is a good summary here of the putative properties of gemstones. Thus, amethyst helps communication and with stomach problems. Aquamarine is good for grief. Carnelian stopped her hubby's allergies. This site offers an elementary education on chakras. "Over time," she informs us, "these points can become clogged from stress, anxiety or improper diet. The Chakras can unclog by meditating with the gemstones...." At the very worst, you'll buy some pretty, if slightly overpriced, jewelry.

By the way, there's a cranky critique of the crystal craze by a professional skeptic named Robert Todd Carroll:

http://wheel. ucdavis.edu/ ~btcarrol/ skeptic/crystals.html

HEALTH
NEWS
NATURALLY

http://www.keats.com/news/index.html

This magazine is published free of charge
in both print and online versions, by Keats Publishing,
one of the pioneers in health publishing in the US.
It contains lots of interesting info
on new developments in prevention.

Nathan Keats is one of the pioneers of the health publishing industry. He left a job at a mainstream New York publisher many years ago to start publishing books on more natural approaches to health. He got into this long before such topics were so trendy.

This Keats Publishing site is both clean and attractive. The articles—and they are real articles or meaty book summaries—are informative, well-written and grounded in the medical literature. I was particularly impressed by "Estrogen: Its Rewards and Its Dangers: Restores Youth? Or Boosts Cancer Risk?" by Dr. Ronald Klatz and Dr. Robert Goldman. The doctors are authors of "Stopping the Clock," not surprisingly a Keats title.

At the end of the article they offer up half a dozen resources to contact for further information. These range from mainstream groups to a service you can call that offers phone consultations with nurse practitioners who will "discuss herbal remedies and natural hormone treatments for menopause as well as conventional hormone therapy."

If you are confused about food supplements this is a good site to visit. Look at the doctor's column. For example, in one of these, Health News Naturally asked prominent nutritional scientists, "Which supplements do you take—and why?"

Denis Miller, MD, an oncologist, reported:
"I don't smoke, get plenty of exercise daily, try to maintain a low (less than 20 percent) fat, high fiber diet, avoid cured foodstuffs, and savor the 'Mediterranean diet,' with its high intake of fresh fruits and vegetables, pasta and wine in moderation.

He goes on. "The hypothesis that beta-carotene would prevent lung cancer has been challenged seriously in recent, highly publicized studies. It may be that other non-nutrient components in fresh fruits and vegetables, and not beta-carotene, are the key anticarcinogens. Citrus fruit oil contains the monoterpene d-limonene, and tomatoes are a rich source of lycopene; both are potent anti-carcinogens. Red wine contains quercitin and epicatechin, flavonoids which reduce LDL levels and salicylic acid which decreases the risk of myocardial infarction. I also take 65 mg of aspirin daily.

"To supplement my dietary intake of these proposed anti-carcinogenic components, I take a daily multivitamin/mineral complex that contains 100-200 percent of the RDA for standard vitamins and minerals, plus vitamin E (400 IU) and selenium (200 mcg). I can also confirm that 40 drops daily of the herb extract of the Eleutherococcus senticosus maxim root, a relative of Siberian ginseng, adds to my sense of general well-being."

This is sensible advice. Personally, I would skip the aspirin and possibly increase my intake of garlic or fish oil. But I always feel better after visiting this site: it reassures me that not everything in alternative medicine is entirely speculative or even wacko.

You definitely get the feeling that sensible people believe in these approaches and derive reasonable benefit by doing so.

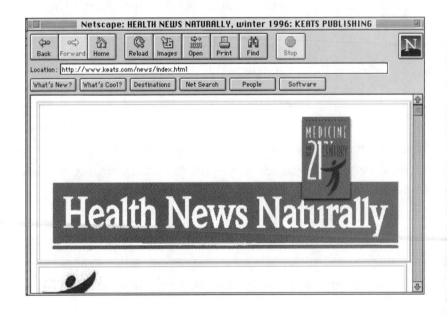

HERBALGRAM

http://www.herbalgram.org/

This is the Web site of three inter-related organizations.
They are the American Botanical Council;
the Herb Research Council; and HerbalGram magazine.

The American Botanical Council (ABC) was founded in November 1988 as a nonprofit education organization. Its main goal is to teach the public about beneficial herbs and plants. The ABC puts out HerbalGram, which is edited by the always amusing Mark Blumenthal. It is supported in this effort by a sister organization, the Herb Research Foundation. It's a rather complicated set of relationships, negotiated with all the delicacy of international diplomacy. The important point is that they put out what is certainly the loveliest publication in the field of alternative medicine, HerbalGram.

This is an outstanding site created by an outstanding constellation of groups and individuals. They have raised medical herbalism in the United States to a new level of probity and respectability.

ABC says that their goal is to "disseminate factual, accurate information on herbs and herbal research. Increase public awareness and professional knowledge of the historical role and current potential of plants in medicine. Contribute information to professional and scientific literature that helps establish accurate, credible toxicological and pharmacological data on various types of plants and plant materials." The organization also promotes understanding of the importance of preserving native plant populations in both temperate and tropical zones.

It thus provides an important link to the environmental movement. It provides reprints of historic plant-related articles, audio/video tapes, and other educational materials. Finally, it assists the aforementioned Herb Research Foundation in achieving its goals.

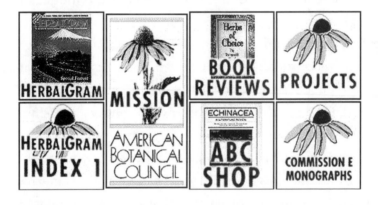

HerbalGram is perhaps unique in another way: it is simultaneously a peer-reviewed scientific journal and a lusciously illustrated book, a sort of Smithsonian for herb lovers. I have enjoyed reading this periodical for years and watching it grow.

The HerbalGram Web site, sad to say, is somewhat less satisfying than the print version. Perhaps that is inevitable, since screen resolutions cannot equal those of four-color printing. However, I do not think that the site contains enough herbal research itself.

Most everything here is for sale. I understand that people have a need to make a living. But wouldn't it be better to allow people to download some of the rich information these experts have gathered over the years? Many experts believe that content-rich sites actually make good economic sense, since people are more likely to buy books that they have at least sampled on the Internet.

That said, you should expose yourself to HerbalGram and its parent organizations. Unless you've already immersed yourself in the world of herbal medicine, you can hardly imagine the treat in store for you.

HERB GARDEN

http://www.nnlm.nlm.nih.gov/pnr/uwmhg/

One of the most pleasant days I have spent since childhood
was a lazy afternoon in the medicinal herb garden
at the University of Washington. Imagine my surprise at finding
this garden reproduced at the U of W's "cybercampus."

The University of Washington houses the largest medicinal herb garden in the Western Hemisphere. This educational and amusing site offers a computerized tour of that garden. From the start, it cautions visitors: "Before we begin, please bear in mind that this garden is the work of many volunteers. Please respect their good intentions. Pick up your cigarette butts and candy-wrappers. Dispose of them properly. Leave only virtual footprints as you explore this aromatic reserve. Please do not look for or exchange medical advice on the premises. Just listen to the plants."

Very amusing. They explain that "your virtual footsteps will take you on a path that exists only in cyberspace. Which is to say, when you visit the real Medicinal Herb Garden... you will find things are a bit more complicated than they might appear here.... Nevertheless, the images presented here may give you a taste of the riches that are stored in these scant hectares of real estate...."

There are indeed riches here, which can brighten the bleakest afternoon spent sitting at a computer terminal. The site offers a walking (i.e., photographic) tour through this lovely garden as it was in 1994 when I visited it. It also offers several charming winter views.

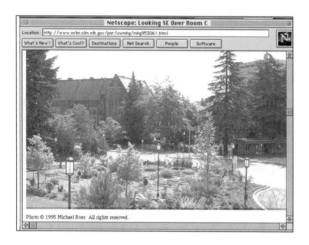

But the site is useful, too. There are excellent indices, categorized by both botanical and popular names, of approximately 100 plants that have been photographed. These represent only about 10 percent of what the physical garden contains. The photographs, by Michael Boer, are aesthetically pleasing and instructive. The headings of each picture gives the natural range of the plant and its location in the physical garden, in case you are planning a visit.

There is nothing like an afternoon stolen from work and spent in a beautiful botanic garden. But if you can't get away, this is the next best thing. And if you ever wondered what "Angel's Fishing Rod" looked like, or where you are likely to find the Cardinal Monkeyflower, this is definitely the site for you. But be sure to clean up after yourself...and don't pick the flowers.

HERPES

http://users.quake.net/~xdcrlab/hp/herpes.html

This Herpes Alternative Approaches site won't win any awards for beauty. But behind its plain facade there lurks a content-rich site that could help those dealing with a tragic health problem.

The articles at this herpes site tend to be long, fact-filled, well referenced, and somewhat on the dull side. This is not a commercial site, and thus is able to give independent information. You do not feel pressured to buy a "cure" or subscribe to some philosophy or ideology here. Just the facts.

Topics covered include the Basics of herpes infection, some alternative treatments, how to practice safer sex, herpes testing, what is called "Herpes Techno/Science," social support links, Newsgroups, Mailing Lists, Health Links, and a grab bag category called Anything Goes.

Naturally, the area that interested us the most was the Alternative department. There are about two dozen such treatments listed. One that I knew a little bit about was transfer factor (TF), an intriguing idea first proposed in the 1940s at New York University.

The writeup of the work of pioneer TF researcher Dr. Hugh Fudenberg was good. They also offered access to his video tapes, something I had never seen before. This made me appreciative of the completeness of this site.

I also was excited by the discussion of Red Marine Algae, which also was the subject of an informative write-up. There was information about such treatments as olive leaf extract, uño de gato (Cat's Claw), the Venus Fly Trap (Carnivora) treatment, etc. The writeup on Thymic Peptides on the other hand was mainly negative.

Naturally, I also liked the "Anything Goes" section, which contained some of the really far-out treatments (Red Marine Algae being practically orthodox medicine in some people's book).

What I liked most about this site, however, was that it looked at the disease from the patient's perspective. The authors/Webmasters are fighting the infection themselves, have tried some of these treatments, and are very frank about their experiences. They are open-minded, and also skeptical, but not to a fault. In other words, intelligent folk who expect their readers to be equally intelligent.

The Herpes site is a potential life-saver for those with this common but persistent infectious disease.

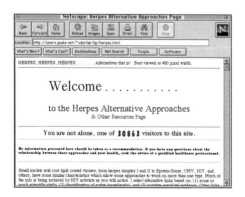

HOMEOPATHIC EDUCATION

http://www.homeopathic.com/

This is a commercial but very educational site. The Homeopathic Education Services describes itself as "North America's LEADING resource of homeopathic books, tapes, medicines, software, correspondence courses, and general information on homeopathy."

This site is the creation of an indefatigable publicist of homeopathy, Dana Ullman, MPH, of Berkeley, California. Dana has been energetically promoting the understanding and use of homeopathy for decades. He is a leading author in the field, and his Web site has the same degree of clarity and organization as his many books and tapes. It is an attractive and well-organized site.

Not surprisingly, there is a great selection of valuable and well written information here. For example, under "Introduction to Homeopathy," one finds all of the following:

Common Questions About Homeopathy • **An Introduction to Homeopathy:** A Modern Perspective • **The History of Homeopathy,** With More Detailed Reference to Homeopathy in America • **The Present Status of Homeopathy Internationally**

• What Connection Do Homeopathic Medicines Have to the Immune System • What Are the **Limits and Risks** to Homeopathic Medicine? • **Homeopathic Constitutional Medicines:** Bodymind Personalities • The Interface Between Homeopathic and Conventional Medicine

From the "Interesting Stuff" section I learned that there are references to homeopathic principles in the Bible. I also learned the origin of the doctor's symbol, the caduceus. In Numbers xxi it states that as a cure for snakebite, "Moses made a serpent of brass, and put it upon a pole, and it came to pass, that if a serpent had bitten any man, when he beheld the serpent of brass, he lived."

I learned that Mother Teresa's clinics dispense homeopathic medicines to the Indian masses. ("At present," writes Ullman, "four charitable homeopathic dispensaries are run under the guidance of the Mother's Missionaries of Charity....several Sisters are studying homeopathy at a homeopathic medical college in order to improve the care they can offer poor people.")

This significant fact has somehow eluded 99 percent of the writers who have commented on this charitable work. There is even humor here: in a spoof, I even learned how Superman could cure his "allergy" to kryptonite with "a highly dilute dose of kryptonite." This produced a homeopathic dose of laughter.

There are numerous homeopathy related sites online. You might also look at the following:

http://www.dungeon.com/~cam/homeo.html

IBIS

http://www.teleport.com/~ibis/

The Interactive BodyMind Information System:
A clever title and a good idea. It is managed by AMR'TA,
the Alchemical Medicine Research and Teaching Association,
a non-profit organization dedicated to reuniting
the art of healing and the science of medicine.

We have spoken before about AMR'TA's own Web site. In addition, these energetic folk (who prefer to remain in the background) also manage the busy Paracelsus newsgroup. Another thing they do is manage the IBIS Web site.

The IBIS site is not to be confused with the complete computerized IBIS data base, which was created a few years ago. This huge project is supposed to give you the—pardon the oxymoron—"standard alternative" treatments for almost any disease. You feed in a particular complaint, wait a minute or two, and out pops a huge and comprehensive description of treatments found in various health systems around the world—actually, those found in standard texts from around the world. The cost of the complete IBIS program is many hundreds of dollars.

I wouldn't bother mentioning this if it weren't for the fact that the IBIS site gives a generous sampling of their wares on the Internet.

So these sample printouts can be helpful for anyone involved with the following medical problems: **asthma** • **benign prostatic hypertrophy** • **bronchitis** • **cystitis** • **hypertension** • **hypoglycemia** • **low back pain** • **menopause** • **osteoporosis** • **peptic ulcer disease** • **premenstrual syndrome** • **rheumatoid arthritis** • **vascular headache**

Nothing I have said so far could prepare you for the extent of the data they provide. Let us take, for example, the first disease listed above, asthma. First they give a succinct definition and etiology of the ailment. These are accurate enough, although most of it could have come out of the Merck Manual. They then follow this with various treatment suggestions, which are definitely not medicine according to Merck. These suggestions cover over 30 pages, single spaced at that, and range from mild aerobic exercises, especially swimming, to astrology and theotherapy. Theotherapy—it's not in my Webster's, but it sounds suspiciously like prayer to me. I guess theotherapy might be tried for any intractable condition.

In between, you will find detailed instructions on hydrotherapy (including something called "garlic hot water" to deal with acute attacks); manipulation, and I assume they refer to the physical and not the psychological kind; electrical and oscillating treatments; dietary principles; therapeutic foods to "tonify the Lung Yin," fresh juices, including a particularly pungent lime, horseradish and garlic drink; and what they call specific remedies.

These specifics might be well grounded in the medical practices of other cultures, but look funny isolated from their holistic contexts. Thus, a "specific" for shortness of breath is steamed salmon three times per day. Walnut kernels, mashed peaches and rehydrated persimmons are some of the other treatment suggestions.

But this is just the beginning. They have combed the world alternative literature to find psychosocial explanations as well. Asthma, they say, may be "related to struggles for independence from maternal influence" or the result of "emotional conflicts between the parents and siblings..." Well, maybe. If you're not sold on the Freudian take, they also include some Jungian interpretations to round things out.

I found the suggestions here a bit overwhelming. Which do you do first—poach the salmon, grind the horseradish or excoriate your mother? But this is a thorough and scholarly effort, and you will soon know more about the above-mentioned diseases. But you get through reading such a list and find yourself longing for the simplicity of a quick cure.... From such lazy impulses is old-fashioned quackery born. And the Internet is the perfect place to satisfy such revisionist yearnings.

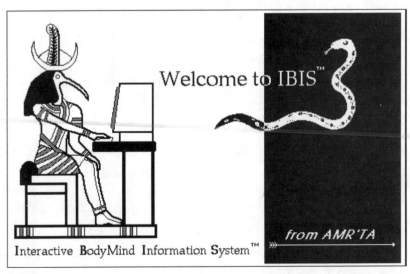

IMAGERY

http://www.electriciti.com/atlantis/

Atlantis: The Imagery Newsletter, has given up
paper-and-ink publication
and launched itself on the turbulent waters of the Internet.

I generally avoid all sites with the word 'Atlantis' in the title. Call me narrow-minded, but as far as I'm concerned, what's actually known about the famous Lost Continent is contained in two small passages in Plato's Timaeus and Critias. However, this site—despite the title—seems to be only tangentially connected to lost, sunken or exploded continents. It is in fact a serious effort by a physician, Dennis Gersten, MD, to educate his colleagues and patients about the tremendous power of visualization. And Dr. Gersten is both passionate and articulate on the subject.

"The main focus of Atlantis is on health and wellness," he writes. "The remaining 20 percent of our newsletter teaches you about sports, Olympic mental training, business, creativity, education, and spirituality. Just twenty years ago," he reminds us, "the importance of exercise and nutrition were entirely underestimated by our [medical] profession. Yet look what's happened. Exercise and nutrition moved to an undisputed central position in good health. Mental imagery is in the same position today...." A good point, made in an nonconfrontational way.

Dr. Gersten quickly had me convinced that the mind and spirit were integral to healing. One of the most attractive things about this mind-over-matter approach to health is its simplicity and, let's face it, the economy. Mental imagery (like its cousin, prayer) is a natural resource that is available at no cost to all of us.

The doctor gives an example of what he means by visualization:
> "Without even closing your eyes imagine you are in your kitchen. Go to the refrigerator. Grab the cold door handle and open the refrigerator. Listen to the hum of your refrigerator. Take out a lemon and smell it. Is it ripe and a little soft...or a little too hard? Either way pick up a sharp knife and go ahead and cut the lemon in half and then in half again. Take that lemon slice and bite into it."

It gives me the shivers! What I especially liked about this site is the emphasis on such simple and homey methods of visualization.

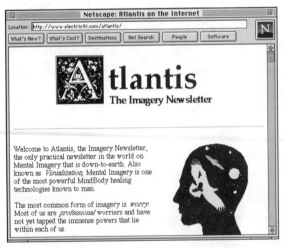

This Atlantis site also contains articles from back issues of the erstwhile printed magazine that could come as a revelation to some readers. Look for instance at Dr. Larry Dossey's outstanding contribution on the relationship of prayer and healing, which was later popularized in his books, such as Healing Words. Here is what Dr. Dossey writes about the so-called Spindrift Foundation experiments, which seemed to show efficacy to third-party prayer:

"The most powerful method of prayer is when the person uses a non-directed approach in which he or she does not attempt to tell the object of prayer specifically what to do., i.e., if he or she prays that 'Thy will be done' or 'May the best thing happen.' This 'let it be' method is difficult for many people to accept, for we usually prefer a directed form of prayer in which we tell the universe what to do—praying for the cancer to go away, the heart attack to repair itself, etc. But the Spindrift experiments show that, although both methods work, the non-directed approach is much more powerful than the directed method."

Many scientifically trained people will of course have difficulty with the concept of any prayer working, either "non-directed" or "directed." Scientists look for mechanisms, and this one seems way beyond the ken. For some religious readers, it will offend in another direction: as Westerners we are used to striking deals with our Deities—just look at Homer, where the odor of roasted flesh is the common coin of prayer. This "I'm-okay-whatever-you-throw-at-me" attitude is likely to come as something of a shock.

That's the beauty of this site. It gets your mind working, which is what imagery is all about. My only criticism is that technically, this site could use a serious makeover. It looks amateurish and the lack of organization makes it difficult to navigate. But these are minor reservations in an otherwise stimulating resource.

KOMBUCHA

http://www.bawue.de/~kombucha/english.html

To qualify as "alternative medicine," a treatment should be exotic, unusual, in fact downright funky. Kombucha tea fulfills all of those criteria, and therefore deserves its craze.

The use of Kombucha spread slowly from the mysterious Far East to Russia at the turn of the twentieth century. I learned here that returning veterans from World War One's Eastern Front brought it further West and in Weimar Germany it was marketed as "Mo-Gu" or "Fungojapon."

In America, Kombucha took longer to catch on. But catch on it did. In the summer of 1993 veteran sensational journalist Tom Valentine wrote about it in his tabloid-style magazine, Search For Health. Against all expectations, this started a prairie fire, a major national health craze, which was eventually noticed—mirabile dictu—by the New York Times.

Since then use of this ancient fermented beverage has spread all over the United States. You can usually tell what's "hot" by looking at the hastily scrawled signs in health food store windows. So judging by that index, "We've Got Kombucha!" has now yielded to "We've got DHEA!" But kombucha has become an established part of the health food scene.

You still might want to check it out and this is the place to do so. The Kombucha Journal shows sufficient fanatical devotion to its product to be included in any comprehensive roundup of alternative treatment sites.

So, down to details. What is Kombucha? It is an old folk remedy made by fermenting tea with a special type of growth. "The Kombucha culture looks like a white rubbery pancake. It is a symbiotic culture of yeast and other microorganisms. The culture is placed in sweetened black or green tea and turns the tea into a sea of health-giving acids and nutrients." (Remember, I'm quoting here.) "The Kombucha culture feeds on the sugar and, in exchange, produces other valuable substances which change into the drink: glucuronic acid, glucon[ic?] acid, lactic acid, vitamins, amino acids, antibiotic substances, and other products. The Kombucha culture is, therefore, a real tiny biochemical factory."

If the thought of eating "rubbery pancakes" makes you drool, you are definitely a candidate for the Kombucha subculture. This site is the brainchild of one Günther Frank, Mr. Kombucha, whose "Persönliches" column reveals that he was born in 1939 in the Sudetenland, Germany and now lives in Berkenfeld. He even gives a picture of Berkenfeld. Mr. Frank has translated instructions for making kombucha into a dozen languages, including Esperanto and Hebrew.

It is sometimes said that alternative medicine is a big ripoff. Skeptics will point out that the altruistic Mr. Frank is also promoting a Kombucha book. Yet to his credit he gives very detailed and reasonably easy-to-understand instructions on how to prepare the Kombucha culture and brew yourself up quarts of the stuff. So this has to be one of the least expensive treatments out there. A panacea in a bottle. Whether it works for anything in particular is another matter. Many people think that it does. Here is a comment from a doctor in Iran, as reported by Mr. Frank: "I distributed the Kombucha among patients. They got good results and are very satisfied. Kombucha was good for Prostate gland, Corns in toes, Rheumatoid Arthritis, Marrow Cancer, Fibroid in uterus, Fibrosis in lung, and so on. I did not hear any complaint about the Kombucha. The results of using the Kombucha were good enough to accept it as a perfect therapy."

Corns and Cancer. This is the kind of thing that generates wet dreams at the FDA of a giant "quackdown" on health food stores selling such products. Luckily, Kombucha went out of fashion before the FDA could swing into action.

There are also horror stories circulating about the dangers of mold contamination and worse. There is said to be an especially great danger in immune-compromised people, such as those with HIV infection, some of whom fell for Kombucha big time. Mr. Frank provides what seemed to me to be commonsensical instructions on molds and such. But if you are seriously concerned about this topic you would do well to search further than this advocacy site.

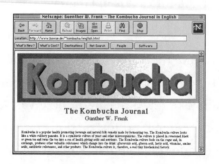

MACROBIOTICS

http://www.macrobiotics.org/default.html

The Macrobiotic diet is very well-known.
This site is one of the many branches of the far-flung
Michio Kushi empire. It is well laid out and contains information
on scientific studies of the diet, as well as patient anecdotes.

Macrobiotics is another fascinating phenomenon. It is both a cause and an effect of the growing American interest in alternative (particularly Asian) approaches to health. Yet at the same time, it is a savvy organization, which knows how to turn a buck.

At this site you will find their trademark mixture of science, faith and high finance. There is much of value in the macrobiotic approach. Take the question of menopause. "Recent studies have shown that grains, beans, and soyfoods such as tofu contain phytoestrogens...mild estrogen-like compounds that act like estrogen in the body. These phytoestrogens can help relieve menopausal symptoms caused by estrogen deficiency."

This is true. A friend of mine was suffering terribly with hot flashes and other menopausal symptoms. She experienced total relief soon after she started eating more tofu and other soy products. And apparently this is not a rare event. Anthropologists have reported that there are not even words for "hot flashes" in

Japanese. And so I do not doubt that this macrobiotic diet can help many people, with menopause or other problems.

As to cancer, there is certainly a lot of evidence to show that elements of the macrobiotic diet are preventive against the Big C. Whether they are curative or not is a big topic of debate.

At this solid site you will find different, sometimes jarring, layers of information. There is the practical stuff on how to prepare rice and beans. There is the grandly philosophical:

"By eating macrobiotic food...the individual naturally begins to develop toward universal consciousness and arrive at a deeper understanding of the meaning of life and death."

And then there is this: the Kushi Macrobiotic Company (KMC), a for-profit corporation in Delaware, has made a special presentation to the Wall Street investment community at the Waldorf-Astoria Hotel in New York. "About 250 stockbrokers listened to a forecast of the company's plans and sampled macrobiotic cuisine. Start up funds were obtained by a private and public stock issue. Stock in the company will be traded on the Nasdaq stock exchange, and the opening price is $5.00/share."

Am I the only one who finds these juxtapositions a little weird?

MAGNESIUM

http://www.execpc.com/~magnesum/

Not every mineral has its own home page.
Magnesium does, and boy, what a page it is.

Magnesium to some is simply a light, malleable, ductile metal. To others, it is a cause. They believe that a deficiency of magnesium is a (the?) leading cause of heart disease in the US and the world. In fact, they say that magnesium deficiency may cause 215,000 fatal heart attacks in the US each year (and as many as 20,000,000 world-wide). They also implicate magnesium deficiency in many other diseases and conditions. The solution is to take a supplement or to drink water that is high in magnesium and calcium.

They have some facts on their side, to be sure:
> "According to the US National Academy of Sciences (1977) there have been more than 50 studies, in nine countries, that have indicated an inverse relationship between water hardness and mortality from cardiovascular disease."

According to these scientists, people who drink water deficient in magnesium as well as calcium generally appear more susceptible to this disease. They quote the aforementioned Academy as estimating that a nation-wide initiative to add calcium and magnesium to soft water might reduce the annual cardiovascular death rate by 150,000 in the United States.

This link between magnesium and cardiovascular illness has been known for decades. In 1957, a doctor Kobayashi observed a geographical correlation between stroke-associated mortality and river water acidity. He inferred from this a possible relationship between the composition of drinking water and cardiovascular diseases.

Forty years later most doctors don't know anything about this and care even less. They act as if hundreds of studies haven't been done. They don't realize that drinking "hard water" (rich in minerals) is generally good for their patients and themselves. They don't know that drinking water should never be artificially softened. Or that people should make sure they are getting enough of these vital minerals.

I'm getting into the mood of this site. But I see their point. For if these "hard water" types are right, then a very powerful means of simply and inexpensively preventing many diseases is being tragically overlooked.

This site is maintained by two obsessive fans of magnesium, Paul and Janet Mason. Together, they own Adobe Springs, a bottled water company in western Stanislaus County, California. Adobe Springs claims that its water has the highest magnesium content— 110 milligrams per litre—of any commercially available water in the country. It also has a low sodium content, another plus.

In a sense, then, this is a commercial site. However, that hardly tells the whole story. The Masons are devoted to a cause. Their tone is scholarly to a fault. There are no frills to their presentation.

Just the facts, which are left to speak for themselves.

One peculiarity I cannot help but remarking on. Take a look at the abovementioned URL for this site: it contains the peculiar word "magnesum." Magnesum? It ain't in the dictionary. It looks like a typo. A typo in one's URL is not reassuring. But perhaps someone else had already hogged the address "/ ~ magnesium."

A small point, compared to the overwhelming commitment to the Magnesium Hypothesis displayed here. Consider the devotion of the Masons themselves, who live at the springs with their three children. This is a real California story. The elevation of their home is 1,375 feet above sea level and in this rocky terrain, way east of San Jose, they report, there is no agriculture or industry using insecticides, herbicides, chemicals, no smog, or anything else that could foul the purity of the water.

The area is just a rugged wilderness, too steep even for San Jose developers, so remote that there are no schools. Even the US postal service dares not follow them up there. In their mountain redoubt, the Masons home educate their three children and capture water. In fact, Adobe Springs is so mountainous that no bottling plant can be built up there, and the water has to be trucked out in "doubles" carrying 6,000 gallons per load. The Masons then sell their water to the bottler for three cents a gallon. It eventually becomes "Noah's Spring Water" in the Central Valley or "Majestic Bottled Water" elsewhere. It is available through the mail. I wanted to buy some. But although a case was a reasonable $10.00, I found out that the UPS shipping charge to my home was $25.00 per carton. Thus ended that fantasy.

The Masons' main inspiration is Dr. Mildred Seelig, a scientist who has devoted over 40 years of her life to this single topic. Although she is a conventionally trained scientist, her research area and obsession have brought her willy nilly into the realm of alternative medicine. Dr. Seelig can be compelling on the subject. We met at a conference in Oklahoma in 1991 and spent the better part of an evening chatting. The topic of conversation, not surprisingly, was magnesium. So I can understand the Masons' fascination.

Incidentally, the Masons offer a free Web page to any magnesium researcher, such as Dr. Seelig. Several have taken her up on the offer, such as J.R. Marier of the National Council of Canada and Dr. Jean Durlach of Paris, France. But do not anticipate any stampedes. Humanity has a yen for the exotic, and sometimes the simplest solutions (like water) are the ones most easily overlooked.

MAHARISHI U.

http://www.mum.edu

Ayurvedic medicine is making inroads
in the United States. And the Maharishi is once
again in the limelight.

In India, alternative medicine is virtually mainstream. There are said to be 550,000 registered Ayurvedic practitioners there—a number equal to the total population of Alaska. In the south Indian state of Kerala this ancient system of healing has been incorporated into a "barefoot doctor" system to shore up their ailing public health system. Gurus (masters) look for the underlying spiritual causes for such "physical" diseases as rheumatism, diabetes, epilepsy and heart conditions. They may prescribe psychic or psychological treatments which might seem irrational in allopathic medicine. Cures are also allegedly brought about by a wide range of herbal palliatives, oil massages, fomentations and steam baths, all delivered at a nominal cost to the patient.

Ayurveda is now beginning to make inroads in the United States, although the number of trained practitioners is still small. One of the most influential schools of Ayurvedic thought in the US is centered in Iowa. For reasons unknown, Iowa has always been a hotbed of alternative medicine. D.D. Palmer founded chiropractic there over a century ago and both Senator Tom Harkin and Rep. Berkley Bedell hail from the Hawkeye state. Iowa is also home to the Maharishi University of Management in Fairfield.

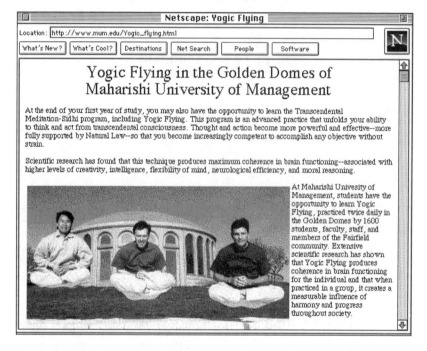

Some people remember the Maharishi as the Beatles' guru. Others think he is the nefarious leader of a brainwashing cult. A visit to this Website might surprise both groups. For along with the inevitable wackiness, there is a considerable amount of scientific sophistication to what the Maharishi followers do.

They all laughed at his trademarked Transcendental Meditation (TM). But this simple system appears to have considerable merit. If you doubt, check out the bibliography of 500 scientific studies on the physiological, psychological, and sociological effects of the method. There is some truth in the TM claim that it is one of the most intensively studied technologies in the whole field of human development. And not all of these have been performed in Fairfield, either. Reports have come out of Harvard, Stanford and about 200 other universities and research institutions on the virtues of this system.

(See http://www. mum. edu/TM_Research/TM_research_home. html for documentation.)

As to the wackiness: the most sensational aspect of what Maharishi U. promotes is "Yogic flying." According to this site, adherents are enabled to actually get off the ground on their own steam for considerable lengths of time. "At the end of your first year of study, you may also have the opportunity to learn the Transcendental Meditation-Sidhi program, including Yogic Flying," we are told with a straight face. In fact, this method is practiced twice daily in the otherwise unidentified "Golden Domes" by 1,600 faculty, staff and students. This would certainly break up an otherwise monotonous cross-country trip.

Outside observers have described this "flying" as a kind of determined bouncing, but no matter. Imagine coming home on Spring break and entertaining your button-down friends by levitating off the front porch.

Well, make of it what you will. Most germane is their description of the courses included in the Maharishi curriculum. These include the following five categories:

1. Consciousness: "...the most fundamental element missing from modern medicine," they say. But "Maharishi Vedic Medicine provides the technology of consciousness."

2. Pulse Diagnosis, Diet, Herbal Food Supplements, along with Physiological Purification Techniques. Reading the pulse is a common element in ancient medical systems. (What humanity did before MRIs arrived on the scene.) They say that their system of pulse readings indicates the degree of balanced functioning of the system, and this in turn helps identify physiological imbalances which form the basis of disease.

3. Environmental Health: This is not what you expect. It is a kind of "Feng Shui," focused on the orientation and shape of buildings. According to the Maharishi's teaching, "recent scientific research showing that direction and orientation have a profound effect on the brain...."

4. Effects of the Extended Environment on Health: They call this the "cosmic counterpart" of human physiology. According to this site, "internal structures of the body, including the DNA, have been found to reflect the structure of the universe, each having its counterpart in such aspects of the cosmos as the sun, moon, planets, and stars." Some people might call this astrology. Let me meditate on it for a while.

5. Collective Health: Here's another headline grabber. The Maharishi Effect is what occurs when a group of people practice TM in one time and place. It has similarities to what we would call group prayer. "Research studies," says the guru, "demonstrate that these technologies strengthen collective consciousness by generating the Maharishi Effect, a powerful influence of coherence, positivity, and harmony in society." According to them, this idea is "as well documented as any principle of modern social science." (Probably true, but that doesn't say much for modern social science, does it?)

They call this "an effective method of social change that operates from the silent, harmonizing level of the unified field to produce a transformation in the quality of collective consciousness, thereby effortlessly creating coherence on a global scale." Jargon aside, I especially liked the 'effortless' part. Creating global harmony the old-fashioned way is such a drag.

In any case, despite my initial skepticism, I actually found this site well organized and strangely compelling. Looking at the pictures of spanking white buildings and sparkling galaxies, I had the feeling that I would enjoy a month or more at the Fairfield campus, with time out for an occasional Yogic bounce. I wonder if I would come out the same Ralph that I went in. And maybe that's the point.

MICHAEL MOORE

http://chili.rt66.com/hrbmoore/HOMEPAGE/HomePage.html

I can hardly find words enough to praise Michael Moore's Web site. This is what makes the hours of slogging through lousy sites finally worthwhile. The Internet at its best.

A recent survey of herbalists revealed that their favorite contemporary author was Michael Moore. This is not the "Roger and Me" funny man, but an equally amusing writer on things botanical.

I first discovered his books, especially Medicinal Plants of the Mountain West, at the gift shop of U.C. Berkeley's wonderful botanical garden. I was immediately enchanted by his irreverent outlook on all topics relating to herbal medicine. This Web site extends that feeling of joy you get when you discover a really good author.

Michael has provided a potpourri of useful, funny and interesting material. His philosophy is to give it all in an unstinting manner. He is not afraid of shooting his wad. (I would still take a course or a consultation with this guy, and I'm sure that many other readers will agree.)

You will come for a look-see and stay for an afternoon. Here is a partial list of what you will find at this engaging site:

Medicinal Plant Images • Michael is big into pictures of herbs, which are essential for those who want to get out in the field and find and harvest their own herbs.

New Images include 47 summer plant images with thumbnails • Medicinal Plant Images by genus. • Over 700 other high quality images of medicinal plants, arranged alphabetically by genus, with a complete thumbnail index files. • Classic engravings and illustrations of drug plants and herbs • Color illustrations from the National Geographic Society, 1915-1924, which are elegant representations of 136 medicinal plants found in North America. • Pen and ink drawings of Western North American plants by botanical artist Mimi Kamp • An index of all 1,100 + images by both genus and species. • Similarly, an index by North American English and Spanish Names • Links to other sites that contain medicinal plant images (by genus).

Overall, the site contains 120 megs of files and has more than 1,000 visitors per day.

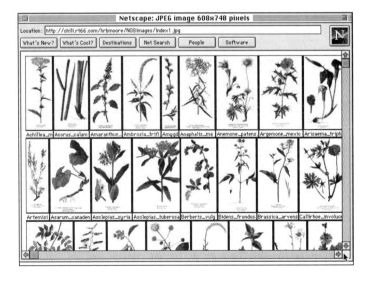

Michael exclaims, "THIS IS FUN!" Vanity publishing? Sure it is. But how many of HarperCollins' writers do you think exclaim "This is fun!" when they ruminate on their careers?

Once again let me express my astonishment over how one determined individual can level the playing field with huge corporations and multi-billion dollar organizations through this remarkable medium called the Internet. Michael Moore's accomplishment is monumental. To add to the wonder, Michael adds "I purchased my first computer 35 months ago at age 53...imagine what YOU could do for our collective benefit!"

Michael has included historical texts and even his own books in both text and Adobe Acrobat format. Yet I doubt very much if his book sales are suffering. With 1,000 visitors per day, that many more people now know about his humorous and well-informed writings. And many of those who come with medical problems will be opened up to the promise of herbal medicine.

NAESSENS

http://www.naessens@cose.com/

This fascinating site gives information about
one of the oddest alternative ideas out there,
the work of Quebec microbiologist Gaston Naessens,
his microscope, condenser, and an unusual product, 714X.

Gaston Naessens is a unique phenomenon. He had no formal education in microbiology or microscopy. Yet he makes claims that seem fantastic by today's standards. He is doing things in both areas that will probably not be recognized for another 50 years.

Naessens is a man of few words. Naturally, there are a lot of people who are happy to speak for him. But this is the authentic voice of his organization, COSE. It is clearly an advocacy and commercial site. (If you want a more objective, scholarly take, see the groundbreaking monograph on his work at the University of Texas website. There are also more popular articles on this treatment in the online Cancer Chronicles.)

In cancer and AIDS circles, Naessens is best known for an unusual medicine called 714X, which contains minute amounts of camphor and mineral salts. These are injected directly in the lymph nodes. Even more provocative is Naessens's work on a class of blood-borne entities called somatids.

These are organisms, if that is the right word, found in the blood of every individual, in fact every living thing that has been examined. They start out as tiny little "blips" in the microscope's field of vision and then apparently transform themselves into different "organisms" in a complicated but definable life cycle.

Reports of such critters date back to the time of the now forgotten Antoine Béchamp in the mid 19th century. Similar reports have come out, over the years, from the laboratories of Virginia Livingston, Gunther Enderlein, Royal Rife, etc.

Do such particles exist? What are they? How come your doctor has probably never heard of this? Well, for them to be seen and studied takes fresh blood viewed under a dark field microscope. (At this site, Mr. Naessens will happily sell you a condenser to help visualize them.) The problem is that orthodox medicine generally does not examine blood fresh, nor does it often have recourse to a dark field. As a general rule, conventional doctors are taught to stain (and thereby kill) blood cells before looking at them, and to examine them under a bright field or possibly an electron microscope. And, as excellent as these are for some purposes, they are inadequate for even becoming aware of the somatid phenomenon.

Seeing is believing and visiting with Naessens made a believer out of me, for sure. I have no doubt that the somatids (and the other weird blood phenomena) are real. Thousands of people have confirmed this. In fact, you would have to be blind not to notice all sorts of bizarre "bugs" dancing around in a drop of blood, especially the blood of sick people.

Scores of naturopaths, chiropractors, and even some MDs use this daily in their work. It is a great discovery, although I am far from convinced that Naessens's own explanation is anything more than a working hypothesis at the moment.

Some conventional scientists dismissively call these particles "artifacts," a word that explains nothing. More sophisticated critics call them "chylomicrons," such as LDL particles. I doubt it. But until someone with knowledge and power starts to take this whole thing seriously conventional science will remain in the dark.

That is why this site is exciting. The Internet will give greater currency to Naessens's theories, and might actually stimulate some good research on this topic.

The Web site is maintained by Naessens's stepsons, who also run a testing and research laboratory in Rock Forest, outside of Sherbrooke, Quebec. The site is multi-lingual, available in French, England and Spanish. I include their site despite the fact that they violate my first rule of Net aesthetics, and include illegible yellow-on-white type.

There are some flashy graphics, and a fair amount of material on 714X, immunity and so forth. There is little visible activity or change at the site itself. (Many people think of the Internet in a static way. Pay someone to put up a site and then forget about it.)

In sum, it's a good site that provides information on a new way of thinking about cancer, AIDS, health, in fact life itself.

NATURAL
HEALTH
VILLAGE

http://www.naturalhealthvillage.com/

The Natural Health Village is the brain child
of Michael Evers, a lawyer-activist
in the field of alternative health rights.

Michael is 110 percent committed to medical freedom of choice.
He is an articulate spokesman for the more militant point of view.
And this is an outstanding site, a real breakthrough in Cyberspace.

The site has been carefully organized, with an eye on the masses
of readers who are coming over from Compuserve and AOL. That
means that they have gone light on the graphics for now.
(Something I forgot when, in my first flush of cyberenthusiasm, I
loaded my site with animated flying unicorns and other fancy
graphics.)

This site, like a number of others, is organized around a New
England "Village Green," with different sections represented by
different buildings. It sounds corny on paper, but I actually found
the format friendly and reassuring. It is divided into three main
sections: "What's New," "The Learning Center," and "Town Hall."

"What's New" contains breaking news (such as updates on Dr. Burzynski trials and tribulations). There are also back issues of the "Natural HealthLine" newsletter, which I will get to in a minute. The section also contains information on a bill in Congress called "The Access to Medical Freedom Act."

What a difference the Net makes! In the past, people would write newsletters containing an article or two about this bill and laboriously send this out to their subscribers.

But Natural Health Village not only can give you their own opinion about the bill (favorable), but can provide the full text of the Senate and House versions, the Hearing statements of Senators Kassebaum, Daschle, Dole, Hatch, etc. on this topic, the Senate testimony of such leaders as Wayne Jonas, MD, director of the OAM, New York physician Woodson Merrell, MD, patient advocate Hon. Berkley Bedell, OAM board chairman James Gordon, MD, as well as opponents from the office of the commissioner of the Food and Drug Administration. So you can be almost as well informed as if you were at the Hearings themselves. It then provides a list of the current sponsors of the bill, with suggested actions.

All of this is laid out in a bright and cheerful format, maybe a bit too slick, but easy to understand and use. To me, this is one of the ways in which the Internet is going to make a difference in the political process. It is going to make online activists a lot more effective! In my moonier moments, I believe this is leading us to a higher level of democracy, at least for those who can venture out onto the Information Superhighway.

Town Hall reduplicates some of the above information, but also gives us the very valuable Senate and House email directories. Just to test it out I searched out a Congressman I knew slightly, typed out a note thanking him for his support of this Bill, and then made some other suggestions and emailed it over to his desktop.

That took two minutes. To be honest, never in a million years would I have taken the trouble to find the right paper, envelope and stamp, and sit down and write a physical note like that. But email and Natural Health Village made it convenient. About two weeks later I received the nicest email back from the guy, too, not just a form letter but a personal note with some valuable information in it. Astounding!

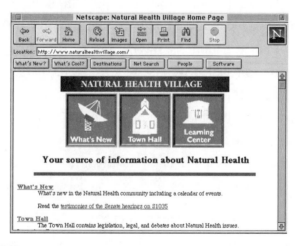

And there's more. They provide readers with a "heads up" on FDA actions, such as the agency's first attempts to regulate the Internet, something of intense interest to paranoiacs like myself.

There is also the "Learning Center." (What does this correspond to in the real world. Does your town have a "learning center"?) This is described as "the largest collection of informational resources related to Natural Health." This is wishful thinking at the moment. But there is much valuable stuff here, including the full text of the government's "Chantilly Report" on alternative medicine (see above). It was left to Natural Health Village to publish this site.

Best of all, Natural Health Village offers free subscriptions to its newsletter, HealthLine®. You send michael@evers.com. an email with the word SUBSCRIBE in the description line or in the body of the message. That's it. HealthLine is published every two weeks and contains articles by Kate White, Peter Barry Chowka, and Mike Evers himself. I very much look forward to this, especially Peter Chowka's commentary. (Peter's own provocative site is at http://members.aol.com/pbchowka/index.html)

NATUROPATHS

http://healer.infinite.org/Naturopathic.Physician/

Naturopathy is on the rise. In April, 1996 Maine Governor King signed the Naturopathic Licensure Bill, making Maine the tenth state in the nation to license naturopathic doctors.

It was also the second state within three weeks to enact such a law. "Naturopathic medicine seems to be on a roll," said commentator Peter Chowka, "experiencing new momentum toward licensure in many more states." If you are not familiar yet with naturopathy, here's a convenient way to check it out.

Real naturopaths, trained at one of the accredited colleges or universities, can be knowledgeable and skillful healers. But because naturopathy is still only licensed in a handful of states, it is especially important to check the credentials of anyone claiming to be a naturopath. There are some phonies out there as well.

A real naturopath attends a four-year graduate level federally accredited naturopathic medical school and is educated in all of the same basic sciences as an MD.

They also receive instruction in holistic and nontoxic approaches to therapy with a strong emphasis on disease prevention and "optimizing wellness."

This site will help you find the real NDs, plus provide a whole lot of other information. It is a content-rich and user friendly place to start any search for alternative medical information.

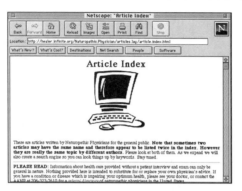

The articles section is one of the plainest sites you've ever seen, but contains a treasure trove of practical material on how to treat a variety of conditions with natural agents. Very solid.

The articles were written by naturopathic physicians for the lay public. Oftentimes, these doctor-authors give their home pages, email addresses and even their phone numbers at the bottom so you can call them. That's quite a departure from the typical medical journal article, where it seems especially important never to reveal the sex of the writers (as in Jones JJ, Smith SS, et al.).

Each of these articles is clearly written, and offers concise and sensible starting points for self-help, as well as accurate medical references for further study. The palpable intelligence of these naturopaths will probably make a convert out of you, especially if you've been "burned" by the cookie-cutter mentality of allopathic medicine. Naturopathy is definitely on the comeback trail.

I could not resist publishing the full list of the subjects covered at this remarkable site:

Acne
Addictions
Aging
Aids Help
Alcohol, Importance in Medicine
Alcoholism
Allergy Relief
Alterative Botanicals
Alzheimer's
Amenorrhea
Anti-Aging
Antibiotics: Sensible Use or Abuse?
Anti Cancer Diet
Arthritis Botanicals
Asthma: A 26 page paper on alternative therapies, Part One
Asthma: A 26 page paper on alternative therapies, Part Two
Asthma in Children
Baby's Health
Bladder Infection Treatments
Breast Cancer Prevention: The role of Fiber and Fat
Breast Cancer Prevention
Breasts: Health and Prevention
Cancer: Prevention
Cancer Botanicals
Cancer: A Complementary approach
Canker Sores
Carpal Tunnel Syndrome
Cardiovascular Botanicals
Chinese Medicine
Cholesterol
Coffee: America's Favorite Drug
Cooking with Grains
Cooking with Greens
Common Cold
Colds & Flus
Colds: Chinese Herbs
Computer Eye Strain
Coughs; many remedies
Coughs, treatment with Herbal Remedies
Compassionate Self Care
Detoxification
Diabetes: Adult Onset

Diabetes Botanicals
Ear Infections: Otitis Media Facts and Treatment
Ear Infections: Fact Sheet
Eczema & Dermatitis Botanicals
Enzymes: The Difference Between Raw and Cooked Foods
Eye, Ear, Nose, and Throat Botanicals
Family Medicine Botanicals
Fasting
Fats: Tips for Decreasing
Female Reproductive Botanicals
Fibrocystic Breast Disease
Fever as Healer
Fish: Benefits of eating it
Food Allergies: Case History
Food Allergies
Gall Bladder Botanicals
Grains
Handling the Holidays Healthfully
Headaches and Migraines
Health Care Costs— An Alternative Medicine Perspective
Head Colds
Heartburn
Heart Disease
Herpes
Homeopathy
Homeopathy for Sports Injuries
Hydrotherapy
Hyperactivity and ADD
Hypertension (High blood pressure)
Immune System Support
Immunity: Building Your Immunity Now
Infants: Prevention of Food Allergies With Proper Timing of Solid Food Introduction
Infertility
Insomnia
Juices
Lead in Grapefruit
Lead in Children
Liver Botanicals
Lower back pain and Acupuncture

Melatonin: A Look at the Research
Menopause
Menstrual Cramps
Migraines
Multiple Sclerosis and Alternative Medicine
Natural Supplements
Obesity: Finding right diet
Osteoarthritis
Osteoporosis
Osteoporosis: Caffeine, Sugar, and Bone Loss
Pain Botanicals I
Pain Botanicals II
Pap Smears: Natural Treatments for Abnormal
PMS: Pre-Menstrual Syndrome
Parent Health Rights
Prostatic Disease
Poison Oak: Protection
Prescriptions for Healthy Traveling
Pregnancy: First Trimester Nausea
Prostate problems
Psoriasis
Rashes
Repetitive strain injuries
Serotyping and Diet— D'Adamo Serotype Panel
Sinusitis
Sore Throat
Sports Injury prevention
Stroke
Sugar
Summer Bugs and Bites
Teething
Tendonitis & Bursitis
Top Nine Calorie Foods in the American Diet
Uterine Fibroids
Vaginitis
Vitamins & Minerals— How Much is Enough ?
The Wai'anae Hawaiian Diet
Walking, the best exercise
Weight Loss strategies
Weight Loss: Mineral that Helps
Weight Loss: The Ten Commandments
Winter Blues

NUTRITION

http://deja-vu.oldiron.cornell.edu/~jabbo/index.html

A wealth of information about diet and nutrition,
divided into three sections:
Current Topics, Just the FAQs, and Some Links.

The Cornell-based locale is not only informative, but humorous and open-minded, qualities you appreciate when you have to review thousands of ho-hum sites. One problem is that we are never told who the overly modest Webmaster is. S/he identifies him/herself as the mysterious "tjt3" at cornell.edu.

Current Topics is essentially an open forum: "The essays collected here are presented for your consideration, not because I agree with them or endorse them, but because they ought to make you think. And it seems like people have been thinking much less these days." Basically, anyone can upload an article here, and so the quality (and sanity) varies greatly. Some of the topics here:

Poisonous Plants? • Magnesium in Your Water • Food Safety and Health Care Issues • Amputees and Powerlifting • The Great Saturated Fat Scam • Aspartame and Neurotoxicity • Notes on a Vegan Lifestyle • Militant Vegetarianism • Myths About Milk • The Future of Conservation Biology

I checked out the article on "aspartame and neurotoxicity," a topic which is discussed elsewhere in this book (see discussion of the Aesclepius site).This discussion contained some new information, but I was surprised at the vehemence of the argument. I'm as much against artificial sweeteners as the next guy, but was shocked to discover that there are people who believe that aspartame causes senility, blindness, death...the list goes on.

Another rant blames all of our ills on milk. Plain old, never-outgrow-the-need-for milk. Most of us think that common sense dictates that milk couldn't be all that bad. But this site contends that "common sense is often heavily influenced by advertising." Dairy advertising, in this case.

So...are these people nuts? Or have they seen behind the veil of lies woven by Big Business? You will have to decide for yourself. The nice thing is that because of the Internet you can. Having access to this kind of information is just great. I hope the Internet will never be "sanitized" to the point where this is unavailable.

The Frequently Asked Questions (FAQ) section is disappointing. It bills itself as "The Official Answers of Sci.Med.Nutrition To Frequently Asked Questions About Diet and Nutrition!" "Sci.Med.Nutrition" is not otherwise identified. Who are they to give "official" answers to anything? Also, the page is accompanied by a huge New York City police badge. Huhn?

There are also three chapters here called basic stuff, lifestyle, and sports nutrition. I didn't find much that was exceptional here. If you are an absolute beginner, you might find it useful.

ONTARIO GUIDE

http://aorta.library.mun.ca/bc/uct/default.htm

A sober and serious look at a large number
of alternative treatments for cancer.
Also useful as a general introduction to alternative medicine.

This very comprehensive "Guide to Unconventional Therapies" was written by an alphabet soup of organizations: the Ontario Breast Cancer Information Exchange Project (OBCIEP), adapted by the Atlantic Breast Cancer Information Project (ABCIP) and funded by Health Canada. It provides public access to a wide range of health and medical information, but is careful not to give medical advice or interpretation.

Again, I will violate two of my ad hoc inclusion criteria: to avoid really ugly sites and to avoid those which contain stupid spelling errors, especially on their home page. First of all, this site is as plain as a Southern Ontario cornfield.

It also contains a real boner: they ask readers to read their "waver." Unless I'm missing an arcane Canadian variant, a "waver" is "the act of wavering, quivering or fluttering" while a "waiver," the word wanted, is "the act of voluntarily relinquishing a known right or claim." And in fact you can't get into this up-tight site until you have passed through their "waver" page.

They also entice you with exciting links which come to a screeching dead end. Thus, they have a page entitled "BC Survivors Speak..." (I assumed they are speaking of "breast cancer" here and not "British Columbia"). But when you click on this you get "HTTP/1.0 404 Object Not Found" A few more of those and I'm outta here.

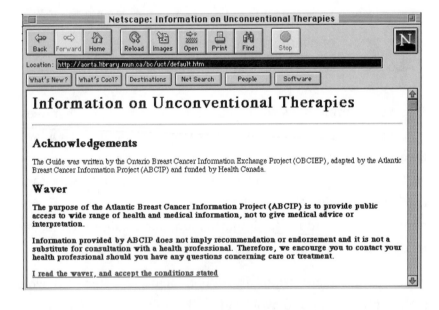

That said, this is an information-rich site. It is in fact the online version of a spiral bound book that was published by the Ontario government a few years ago. Now everyone has access to it for free. It is definitely worth looking into. What they say:

> "We have attempted to bring an open-minded approach to our topic and to avoid either supporting or rejecting particular unconventional therapies."

They warn that no endorsement is intended by the fact that they included therapies in this guidebook. "Nevertheless," they state, "we consider it important for cancer patients who wish to participate in decisions regarding their own treatment to have access to information." This puts them head-and-shoulders above their counterparts to the south, especially the NCI. The OBCIEP sees its role as a catalyst within the cancer control system. "It is our hope that the production of this guidebook will mark the first of a series of initiatives related to unconventional therapies."

A noble goal and an excellent resource.

OSTEOPATHIC MEDICINE

http://www.rscom.com/osteo/

A form of "allopathic" medicine that borders on the alternative.

Does osteopathic medicine belong in a book about alternative medicine. Nowadays, mainstream osteopathy is part of establishment medicine and DOs are almost as respectable as MDs. It was not always that way. The philosophical principles of osteopathy are similar to those of chiropractic, which it helped spawn.

Osteopathy wasn't always a junior partner to the allopaths. Originally, as founded by Andrew Taylor Still (1828-1917), it was an alternative vision of health care based on his theory that:

"...the body is capable of making its own remedies against disease and other toxic conditions when in normal structural relationship and has favorable environmental conditions and adequate nutrition. It utilizes generally accepted physical, pharmacological and surgical methods of diagnosis, while placing strong emphasis on the importance of body mechanics and manipulative methods to detect and correct faulty structure and function."

Today, there are young doctors who want to return to the original osteopath path. The online journal "Still Alive" (clever name!) is their house organ. Its goal is to act as a forum for this more alternative brand of osteopathy, the kind that was preached by the lanky founder. It preaches the combined "art of osteopathic manipulation and naturopathic medicine."

In years past, such an upstart group might have received little attention or exposure, to put it mildly. But thanks to the Internet and the changing medical climate, they are now able to reach a wider audience of both doctors and concerned patients who are bound to be interested in a profession that can combine the best of rigorous Western science with a truly native-born American healing art.

An exciting departure.

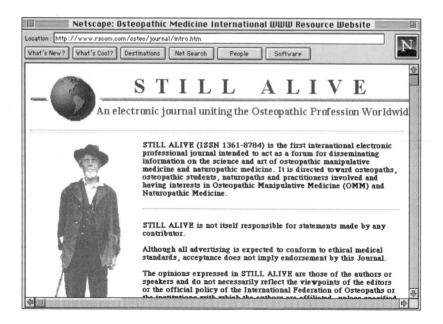

OZONE AND OXYGEN THERAPY

http://www.oxytherapy.com/

Oxygen isn't just about breathing anymore.
This site takes oxygen beyond mere respiration.
They believe that oxygen deprivation in its various forms
is the root cause of all of humanity's ills.

Oxygen isn't just an element. In the hands of some ardent individuals, it is the one true religion. This should generate healthy skepticism about the exaggerated claims sometimes made for Ozone and Oxygen Therapy

Simple and natural approaches to complex medical problems are intrinsically appealing. They rarely come true, but they are so important that they deserve serious consideration. Thus, although I don't know if oxygen therapy really works, it is worth studying.

This is a good place to start. It is a popular and well-organized site "dedicated to the advancement of Oxygen Therapies." Oxygen Therapies include the use of Hydrogen Peroxide (H_2O_2), Ozone Therapy, Hyperbaric Oxygen, Stabilized Oxygen, and Ionization.

There is a vast amount of information here, good, bad and indifferent. Much of this site is authored by Ed McCabe, who calls himself the "father of oxygen therapies." With no false modesty, Ed describes himself as the "undisputed leading journalist specializing in uncovering the truth about oxygen therapies for the benefit of humanity."

Serious questions have been raised about the advisability of using potentially harmful agents such as ozone or hydrogen peroxide in do-it-yourself therapies. If you are looking for a balanced presentation on the pros and cons, you will not find it at this enthusiastic site. Nevertheless, if you truly want to know the full scope of alternative treatments for some serious diseases you should familiarize yourself with this branch of the movement.

Oxygen therapies are popular and there are some lively forums here. One provides a jumping off point for "Alternative Biomedical Electronics." These are the "black boxes" that so exercise FDA enforcers. If you are interested in the no man's land where medicine and electronics intersect, this is a good place to start.

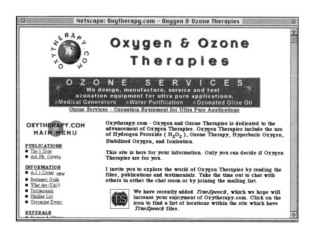

PHYTOCHEMICALS

http://www.ars-grin.gov/~ngrlsb/

American tax dollars at work.
There are five browsable databases here, including
"Medicinal Plants of Native Americans,"
ten years in the making.

These are the Phytochemical and Ethnobotanical Databases of the Agricultural Research Service, USDA. It sounds dull, but this is quite exciting, once you get the hang of the obscure interface. You can search by particular chemicals and their activities, by plants and their uses, and by numerous other categories.

There is enjoyable wackiness here, lurking behind the white lab coat of the laboratory scientist. In what other government database are you likely to find Chinese herbs that are useful in combatting the Evil Eye? This could be very useful in Washington.

This database is another work of genius from James Duke, PhD and his intrepid ethnobotanical colleagues. If you're not familiar with Dr. Duke, this is a good place to start. Jim sort of looks like Burl Ives. For many years, he has been periodically disappearing into the Amazonian rain forest only to reappear with a handful of herbs and astonishing tales of cures in the least accessible places on earth.

He periodically takes well-heeled amateur botanists to his favorite places in the tropics. Jim is both a scholar and a gentleman and has helped create one of the most fact-filled medical databases on the entire Internet.

But be forewarned: this is a very frustrating site to navigate. The presentation should be colorful and dynamic (like Michael Moore's site or the University of Washington Herb Garden.) Instead, I am never quite sure that I am finding what I think I am looking for. You will never forget that you are at the point of confluence of the world's largest government bureaucracy, medical arcana, and plain old IBM obscurantism. Add to that an author (J.D.) who admitted to me that he is virtually illiterate when it comes to computers, and you will understand why you might get a bit confused.

Here are the specific types of inquiries you can perform with these databases:

Plant Searches

Chemicals and activities in a particular plant.

High concentration chemicals.

Chemicals with one activity.

Ethnobotanical uses.

GRIN Accessions.

Chemical Searches

Search for plants with a chosen chemical.

Search for activities of a chosen chemical.

Activity Searches

Search for plants with a specific activity.

Search for chemicals with a specific activity.

Search for chemicals with a lethal dose (LD) value.

Ethnobotany Searches

Ethnobotanical uses for a particular plant.

Plants with a particular ethnobotanical use.

Database References

Reference citations.

To illustrate how this works, let's say you are interested in Morinda citrifolia, a.k.a. noni juice. You go to the Ethnobotany Query, then enter Morinda in the genus and citrifolia in the species box. The database will quickly come up with a long list of indications. This confirms that it is considered a panacea in the world literature. An asterisk indicates that it has been shown to have a particular application in the scientific literature.These are lacking for noni. So you get a quick snapshot of a plant's usage.

Conversely, let's say you are interested in a particular chemical, such as benzaldehyde, but do not know in which plants to find it. A search for "benzaldehyde" yields 16 plants, headed by licorice, whose oil contains 75,000 parts per million of the chemical. Sweet almonds, by contrast, contain only one ninth as much.

The medical and industrial properties of benzaldehyde are also listed, viz., "Allergenic; Anesthetic; Antipeptic; Antiseptic; Antispasmodic; Antitumor; Flavor; Insectifuge; Motor-Depressant; Narcotic; Nematicide; Pesticide; Sedative." And that's just for starters. You can get lost in this incredibly dense Amazonian tangle of obscure data. But if you are interested in herbs in a serious way, you can be thankful that Jim Duke and his friends have hacked their way through the underbrush and brought back these nuggets of botanical knowledge.

PROSTATE POINTERS

http://rattler.cameron.edu/prostate/

Come a certain age,
most men become aware of their prostates.
This site is the first stop in dealing
with all troubles prostatic.

The prostate gland works best as an invisible team player. Once you become aware of it, it means you've got trouble. The most common such trouble is benign hyperplasia of the prostate (BHP). Almost every male gets it in time. The worst is prostate cancer.

Cancer is a mystery, and prostate cancer is a riddle wrapped in a mystery inside an enigma. This excellent site reveals a few of the imponderables about prostate cancer.

• Prostate cancer in the United States is increasing at a tremendous rate. According to a recent medical article found here,
"Despite these statistics, the appropriate treatment for this disease remains controversial." Treatment recommendations ranged from expectant observation to radical prostatectomy, external-beam radiation therapy, and brachytherapy (seed pod implants).

Even the American Cancer Society admits that much of the increase is due to "improvements" in diagnostic techniques. Some improvements, finding cancers that would have remained indolent just a few years before.

• The Prostate Specific Antigen (PSA) is a wonderful test, but it also sometimes picks up conditions other than prostate cancer, and slips up in other alarming ways. This can lead to false alarms.

• A lot of men with prostate cancer can actually get by without any treatment, a procedure poetically called "watchful waiting."

• Doctors can't seem to agree on who those lucky individuals are.

• If you go to a surgeon, he generally recommends surgery. Radiologists generally recommend radiation. Surprised? Often, they will treat you to lectures on the irresponsible actions of their opposite numbers.

• And then there are the alternative doctors who say they can cure prostate cancer without surgery, but with herbs, drugs, microwaves, heat, cold, 714X, prayer, whatever.

Adequately confused? Then this is the site for you, the best site on the prostate gland ever. In fact, if you have serious prostate concerns, it would be worth your while to go out and buy a computer just to be able to access this site!

A prostate operation is going to cost you thousands of dollars, and may mean a loss of both your sexual potency and urinary continence. Please check out all your viable options before you give in to pressure from anyone.

Prostate Pointer Webmaster Gary Huckabay is another one of those heroic individuals who has singlehandedly built a site worthy of some giant institution or medical center. He writes, "It is my intention to provide the Internet community with a full spectrum of information available about prostate cancer and general problems of the prostate. It is not my intention to pass judgment about any information source; all are treated equally." That, in my view, is the key to his success. "It is up to you," he continues, "to carefully weigh the information you find. Good luck in your search."

The site is especially enlivened by the presence of various prostate specialists, fellow Web-aholics who donate their time trying to enlighten the populace. A special mention to Stephen B. Strum, MD, a Los Angeles area prostate specialist who has a strong passion for helping patients in any context.

You will find a chilling section called "Ice Balls," on the techniques of cryosurgery, a treatment modality that involves freezing the prostate with the use of probes containing liquid nitrogen. Brrrr! Another section deals with brachytherapy, i.e., seed pod implants.

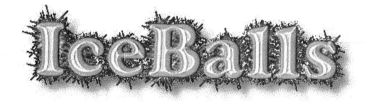

I assure you that an afternoon or two spent at this site will make you, if not an expert, then at least a well-informed medical consumer ready to take on your physician. Imagine your doctor trying to schedule you for a run-of-the-mill radical prostatectomy, and you come out with: "Excuse me, doc, but what is your opinion of formal retropubic exploration through an extra peritoneal lower-abdominal incision, a pelvic lymph-node sampling, and mobilization of the prostate from the surrounding tissues?"

At the very least, that'll get his attention.

QI GONG

http://exo.com/~chi/ch02000.html

Sound for health?
This is the Web site of Infratonic QGM.
Turning Qi Gong into a marketable commodity.

The power of Qi Gong is legendary. Who can forget Bill Moyers' historic conversation in Healing and the Mind with Harvard's David Eisenberg, in which David explains some of the "miracles" of Qi energy he saw while in China?

This energy category is taken for granted in the East, but somehow eludes Western medicine. How scientific is Qi research? Probably more than most Western doctors realize. Experimental subjects include not just humans but test animals as well. (Does a sick parakeet experience placebo effects from applications of Qi?)

You will read at this site that scientists in China have concluded that Qi Gong mediation is either the same thing as low frequency (infrasonic) sound or that the two have similar effects. But warning—this site is also selling low frequency devices, so they might have a reason to present Qi research results selectively.

Qi is another spelling of the more familiar Chi. To add to the confusion, the name of the device in question is Infratonic QGM, but it emits infrasonic vibrations.

Infrasonic sound research originated in Beijing, China, with studies of the abilities of various natural healers. They found—odd as it seems—that some of the most powerful healers "were able to emit a strong infrasonic (low frequency sound) signal from their hands." This theory was subsequently tested in various hospitals and research labs in China which also allegedly found that "infrasonic sound was indeed effective at increasing vitality, accelerating healing, and strengthening immune function."

If you are skeptical about the whole phenomenon, I would urge you to read an enlightening article at this site by Prof. Liu Guo-long. Prof. Guo-long writes:

> "At the beginning of my research with Qi-Gong, I was
> confident that a study of Neurophysiology would prove
> that the 'Wai-Qi' emitted by Qi-Gong masters was noth-
> ing more than a psychological factor induced by the
> waving of hands and hypnotic suggestion....

In other words, placebo. "Up until about 15 years ago," he says, "most Chinese considered Qi-Gong masters...to be mythical story book characters with super-human powers. However, as the Chinese government began to support scientific research into Qi-Gong, the few remaining true Qi-Gong masters began to surface, amazing researchers with feats like killing bacteria in test tubes and causing previously paralyzed people to get up and walk." That would catch anyone's attention, and Chinese scientists are among the most receptive in the world to strange phenomena.

Asthma appears to be one of the diseases most treatable through this low frequency sound method. The site offers a paper by Dr. Su Cheng Wu on 50 cases of childhood bronchial asthma treated by "sub-audible, outgoing qi." Incidentally, Dr. Wu is at the Guangxi Medical University in southcentral China. She reports that "an infra-audible instrument" like the one advertised here has been used to "cure" paroxysmal child bronchial asthma in 50 cases.

Stomach problems—or "Digestive Qi Deficiency" as it is called in China—is another illness being treated with Infratonic QGM.

It surprised me to learn that 7,000 doctors are currently using the device in the United States for soft tissue injuries and pain. Here are some of the soft tissue conditions for which they are reporting some success:

Arthritis pain: home use, applied daily to the arthritic areas as required for pain; substantially reduces consumption of pain medications. **Breaks and sprains:** applied directly over the injury, and where there is a cast, directly over the cast, for 10 to 20 minutes three times a week on high....recovery time is lessened dramatically. **Carpal tunnel syndrome:** applied to the nerve invasion (C7-T1), elbow (if painful) and carpal tunnel area for 10 to 15 minutes on low setting. If pain increases, the applicator is moved a short distance away from treatment area for about 5 minutes and then reapplied to affected area. **Chest congestion:** 10 to 20 minutes on the sternum...often clears out the congestion. **Degenerative or ruptured disks:** applied to the involved disk level for 10 to 20 minutes on high setting to relieve inflammation and swelling. **Inflamed scar tissue:** applied directly over the inflammation on low for 10 to 20 minutes...an immediate reduction in redness and softening of scar tissue. **Menstrual cramps:** used on high setting for 10 minutes along the front line of the body exactly half way between the navel and the pubic bone. A single application is said to be adequate in nearly all cases to stop the pain. **Sciatica:** on high under each foot for 5 minutes. Said to be highly effective. **Sinus headache:** on the eyebrow on medium for 10 to 20 minutes, until the patient feels it clear. Possibly treat the cheeks and below the earlobe as well. **Temporomandibular disorders:** hold the QGM device at the temple, directed downward to the jaw and cheek for 7 minutes on the side that has most pain. Then at the jaw, directed upward from the jaw toward the temple for 7 minutes.

The bottom line to all this is that this is a commercial site. Actually, I was glad about this. One gets tired of reading about "breakthroughs" that are unavailable to the consumer, illegal or only accessible by spending three weeks at a tropical clinic.

Infratonic QGM units cost $695.00, which seems reasonable if the device performs as advertised. I was encouraged by the fact that the company, in San Clemente, CA, offers an unconditional, 30-day money back guarantee to the product. (Of course, be aware that most people will have some placebo relief of pain in the short run, i.e., a month. The real test comes over longer periods.)

Overall, this whole topic of "Qi" energy is one of those exciting new/old areas of medicine. Breakthroughs seem possible for a wide variety of illnesses. Once again, I marvel at this wonderful Internet, which can bring the secrets of Chinese Qi Masters right into our living rooms with a few clicks of the mouse.

QUANTUM MEDICINE

http://www.usa.net/qmed/

Developments in medicine have always been
greatly influenced by those in the "hard sciences," especially
physics and chemistry. But conventional medicine has failed to
make the leap into the mysterium of quantum mechanics.

This site attempts to bridge the gap between 19th century medicine and 21st century physics.

"QMed" provides information on such unfamiliar categories as Quantum Medicine, Electro-Physiological Reactivity including Natural Medicine, Naturopathy, Homeopathy, Bio-Energetics, Acupuncture and Electro–Acupuncture.

The Quantum Medicine site is a truly international effort. It is sponsored by Hippocampus, Inc. which is located in Budapest, Hungary, The College of Practical Homeopathy, in London, England and the Association of Applied Quantum Bio-Technologies, in New Mexico, USA. What they say:

> "The fields of natural medicine, homeopathy
> and energetic medicine have received much attention
> in the last few years. The fear of synthetic chemicals,
> the ecological damage caused by the chemical industry,

failure of antibiotics, realization of the chemical special interest groups ability to manipulate medicine and an overall developing appreciation of nature, all have brought these forms of medicine into our awareness.

"Patent synthetic medicine dramatically profits from its synthetic patents and then tried to get us to believe that the synthetic substance is the same as the natural. More and more people are doubting this."

I want to know more about this perspective. One big reservation about this site is that some of the files are in "zip" format (Word Perfect 6.1), which I cannot download to my Macintosh. But that said, this is an interesting area, and the site is lively and updated frequently. There is enough here that is accessible to all comers to make this site worthwhile and recommended.

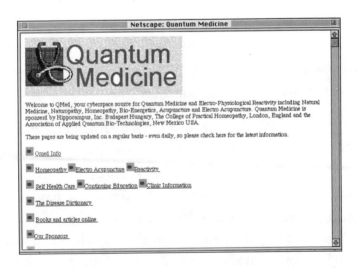

REIKI

http://www.crl.com/~davidh/reiki/

**If you are looking for an energy healing system,
or are just curious about Oriental medicine,
this is a good place to start.**

Reiki is a popular method of natural healing based on the application of what is called the Universal Life Force Energy (said to be a literal translation of the word 'Reiki'). It is one of the vitalistic philosophies that are so popular in alternative medicine practices.

What they say:

> "Reiki is one of the more widely known forms of healing through direct application of Chi [i.e., Qi], or a force very similar to Chi for it may be that Chi is different from the energy used by Reiki. Chi is the term used by the Chinese mystics and martial artists for the underlying force the Universe is made of."

I have friends who swear that they have used this technique to accomplish amazing things. One of the more sensational claims of reiki masters is that they can heal people at a distance, since mundanities such as space and time are actually mere illusions. Another claim is that they can "heal" animals or even inanimate objects.

"Yes, you can Reiki your car!" this Website proclaims. "One trip to

Mt. Shasta I swear the only way we made it to the top was sending Reiki through the gearshift and dashboard into the car." I will be sure to remember this before I take the Subaru into the dealership for an expensive tune-up.

Reiki was developed by a Japanese, Dr. Mikao Usui, who is deeply revered by Reiki's many adherents. This happened some time before World War Two. He said that Reiki is based on a very ancient healing system, although there appears to be little documentation for this claim.

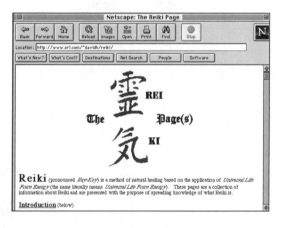

Reiki is also an example of how wildly successful esoteric Asian philosophies can be, especially when the tsunami makes landfall on America's West Coast. Dr. Usui, it is said, taught just one individual, Dr. Chujiro Hayashi, who in turn taught his wife and another woman, Hawayo Takata. Before her "transition," Reiki-ese for death, Mrs. Takata managed to initiate 22 Reiki Masters. These in turn taught others, many others, in well attended seminars. Today, reiki is practiced throughout North and South America, Europe, New Zealand, Australia and other parts of the world.

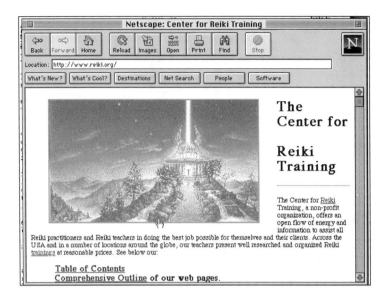

There are now an estimated 5,000 Reiki Masters with as many as half a million people practicing Reiki throughout the world.

To be honest, after reading all about Reiki at this site I still had little idea what it does for you, or what all the excitement is about. But perhaps it is the kind of thing you must experience in order to understand.

See also: http://www.crl.com/~davidh/reiki/history.htm

http://www.reiki.org/

ROSENTHAL CENTER

http://cpmcnet.columbia.edu:80/dept/rosenthal/

Columbia University's Rosenthal Center for Complementary and Alternative Medicine. Its objectives include providing information to practitioners, researchers and the public about alternative and complementary therapies.

The Rosenthal Center is Columbia University's groundbreaking effort to bring alternative and academic medicine together. Located in the Department of Rehabilitation Medicine, and headed by the dynamic Fredi Kronenberg, PhD, the Rosenthal Center specializes in issues of women's health.

This is the content-rich Web site of one of the Office of Alternative Medicine's first grant recipients. This is not only an excellent center but a pioneering effort at bringing sound information on alternatives to the Internet.

This straight-forward and informative presentation is the work of Webmaster Jackie Wootten, who was formerly employed by the Office of Alternative Medicine. I consider it one of the crucial sites for people confronting cancer, and a whole lot more.

At this site you will find descriptions of various projects that the

Center is involved in. One of these is
"Menopausal Hot Flashes: Effect of a Chinese Herbal
Preparation Double-blind, randomized, cross-over,
placebo-controlled trial."

This study will examine, using both subjective and objective parameters, whether a preparation of Chinese herbs is effective as a treatment for menopausal hot flashes. It is surprising that this has never been done before.

This is exactly the kind of study that academic medicine has demanded from alternative medicine over the years. Well, here it is, under the direction of sympathetic, yet rigorous, scientists. Finally we may be about to get some useful and reliable answers.

You've Gotta Be Joking: Alternative practitioners are sometimes accused of clowning around. But now comes a study entitled "Clown Care and Healing" (you can't make this stuff up). This is a serious collaboration between the Rosenthal Center, several prestigious academic departments of pediatrics and that celebrated medical group, the Big Apple Circus.

The point is to assess the impact of the Big Apple Circus's "Clown Care Unit" on the health and well-being of hospitalized children. The studies will soberly quantify the extent to which "laughter, joy, and delight" affect the healing process for hospitalized children, their parents, and caregivers. How do you quantify delight?

On another tack, the Center is conducting literature reviews to determine the state of scientific research in complementary and alternative therapies for breast cancer, nausea and vomiting of pregnancy, breech version in pregnancy, menopausal hot flashes, fibroids, and endometriosis.

Other projects include:

Ethnobotany in the Urban Environment: Herbal Therapies for Women's Health: a multidisciplinary observational study

Complementary and Alternative Medicine Use for Women's Health Conditions: A Multi-Ethnic Perspective

Traditional Chinese Medicine in the Treatment of Uterine Fibroids: An observational pilot study of 25 women

An especially important feature of this site is a comprehensive Directory of Databases, which describes the major databases, worldwide, which have collections on alternative medicine. This is the very best such effort on the Net, and is a tribute to the indefatigable Ms. Wootten, who began collecting these references while working at OAM.

These varied sources of information can seem quite exotic. How about "SIGLE," which is an acronym for the "System for Information on Grey Literature in Europe." SIGLE is produced by EAGLE, which is the "European Association for Grey Literature Exploitation." What does it mean? In Europe, "grey literature" is their term for underground or alternative literature. Yuch! And now it's ready for "exploitation" on the Internet. Somebody should teach these European researchers the nuances of English.

Overall, however, the Rosenthal site is an excellent starting point for any serious, scholarly investigation of alternative medicine, especially as it relates to women's problems.

SELF-HELP

http://cybertowers.com/selfhelp/

This is a content-rich site that is more than just a collection of articles. Well-organized, it feels like a "place" to visit, to find information on a wide variety of psychological approaches to health problems.

To give some idea of the scope of this site, it contains:

A Full Library Covering Over 20 Self-Help Topics

Answers Written by Professionals to Reader Questions

Interactive Zone with Surveys to get Your Opinions

Cartoons and a Meditation Zone with Thoughts and Pictures

Self-Help Search Engine for Our Website

Lists and Newsgroups Spanning Mental Health Sites Across the Globe

Amazing Bookstore Catalog

Professional Zone for Information and Services

Postcards for Your Loved Ones

Distance Learning Classes for You and your Family

Discussion Zones to Meet New People and Write Your Ideas

Self-help offers the reader a chance to send in questions on a wide variety of topics and have those questions answered by experts.

The articles range from the sober and scholarly to the R-rated "Seven Weeks to Sexual Heaven." ("Toss a coin," says author Dagmar O'Conner, PhD. "The winner has the privilege of initiating the first sensuous exercise—of being the one who is touched.")

Self-help's parent group, CyberTowers, sells distance learning courses on the computer. Because of the sensitive nature of some of the material offered, all participants in these courses are anonymous.

"You will be known by just a first name or a nickname or alias. Your email address will not be known to either your instructor or other class participants." Sounds like a wise policy.

Some of these courses are quite unusual. There is one on "Homicide Recovery": which is designed to cover the unique aspects of homicidal death. It includes the psychological aspects of homicide and resources for further study. Another is on Dream Discovery Techniques: From Ancient Thrace to Cyberspace. It offers a wide spectrum of techniques for exploring "the meaning and value of your dream imagery."

You can sign up as a participant in these courses or offer yourself as a potential teacher of these or other courses.

CyberTowers Professional Center, which runs this site, also offers a free email newsletter to those who sign up. CyberTowers is an interesting concept, with which psychologists and other professionals should feel comfortable. I guess their business is selling Websites. But they present them as online 'offices' and the analogy holds throughout this site until you really feel you are in a modern office tower made up of health care professionals. It's a bit hokey but it feels realistic.

What they say:

"From these offices stem multiple services and products that reach throughout the Internet to other professionals, businesses, and clients. Adjunctive businesses are also invited to locate themselves within CyberTowers. Their function will be not only to offer information, services and products to the Global Village, but to neighboring businesses and professionals located within CyberTowers."

SMART DRUGS

http://www.ceri.com/

Smart Drug News is about the pharmaceutical contingent
within alternative medicine. It deals with drugs
that are being used to increase IQ,
and otherwise stimulate the little grey cells.

The site would be very helpful for anyone dealing with cognitive
problems. But what grabbed my attention was the controversy
swirling around one particular drug (or nutrient, take your pick)
called GHB (gamma-hydroxybutyrate).

At this writing, the FDA has banned its sale and the California
legislature is contemplating criminalizing its use. Yet it appears
relatively harmless. GHB is a euphoric, similar in some ways to
alcohol, but without the well-known side effects of booze.

I have no opinion on its value, but I thought this site offered an
extremely well reasoned defense of its potential value, and the
politics of its ban.

The authors plausibly suggest an economic motivation to the
opposition: "In the absence of a genuine public-health concern,
such control might have been motivated by a desire to protect

the pharmaceutical industry (with which the FDA is closely intertwined) from competition from a safer, more effective and less expensive alternative to sleeping pills. Is it a coincidence that the FDA has also banned L-tryptophan, another nutrient that functions as a safe and effective sleep aid?"

I could offer another explanation. GHB sounds like it is pleasurable to take, and there is a large number of people in the population (125 million by my last count) who simply hate anyone to have more fun than they do. They can't do much about the well established vices, but anything new in the fun department is going to run into serious opposition. I wouldn't give GHB much of a chance in this anhedonistic climate.

What they say about themselves:
"Smart Drug News details the latest scientific research in the rapidly growing field of cognitive enhancement technologies and related topics of physical health and well-being, including the latest treatment trends for Parkinson's, Alzheimer's, Down's syndrome, and age-associated mental impairment in normal, healthy adults.

SPIRITUAL HEALING

http://www.spiritweb.org/Spirit/intro.html

Do you believe in spiritual healing? If so, there are many sites on the Web that deal with the effects of spirituality and religion on illness. This is one of the most comprehensive.

SpiritWeb has been online since 1993. It is maintained in Switzerland.

Initially, I found some of the areas on this site off-putting in the extreme. I like to see data in support of claims and assertions. I found the religious-style generalities at such sites quite maddening. Yet I also recognize that science does not have all the answers. It doesn't even have all the questions.

Religion enters areas that cannot be touched by science, and probably always will. So spiritual ideas increasingly resonate with a large number of people. Many such people believe you can harness the power of the spirit to free the body from its physical problems. One good place to start is SpiritWeb or Spirit-WWW, which promotes "spiritual consciousness" on the Internet.

Obviously, not all of this material here is directly related to questions of medicine, much less alternative medicine. Some have more to do with religion or psychology. But if you have medical problems, and especially if you are struggling with an intractable or "incurable" disease, you might want to familiarize yourself with this material. The price is right and what do you have to lose?

This site brings together information of varied quality on a large range of topics. To give you some idea of the depth of content at this particular site, here is a list of its basic categories:

Introduction	Yoga Paths	NewsGateway
What's New	Veda & Dharma	NewsWatch
Channelings	Theosophy	ImageGallery
Lightwork	Mysteries	WebChat
UFO	Astrology	MailingLists
Light Technology	Networks	"Archive"
Healing	Resources	SearchEngine
Reincarnation	Bibliography	
Meditation	Event Calendar	
Out of Body	Glossary	

At the section called WebChat you can have a live conversation with others of a similar spiritual bent. When I went online at around 6 a.m. EST, there were already 11 people talking to one another. They hailed from such places as Sydney, Singapore, Malaysia, Texas and, after I joined, Brooklyn. There wasn't anything particularly "spiritual" about their chat, though. Like most sites, regardless of the alleged specialty, they soon de-differentiate into a kind of universal Cyberchatter:

Roger: "Good Morning Aurora, What a pleasant surprise to see you this early in the morning. Want a cup of coffee? Why are you up so early?"

Aurora: "Mmmm coffee sounds heavenly...couldn't sleep...what else??? I just don't usually come in here this early...will change that if it means talking to you!!!" etc. etc.

Sounds like that obnoxious television commercial of the couple whose illicit love affair is centered around their coffee addiction. Well, perhaps Roger and Aurora will get to the spiritual stuff later.

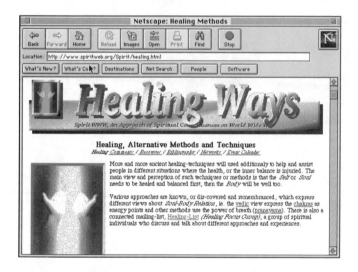

Or here is a sample from the material on the Pleiadians:

"The Pleiadians are a collective of extraterrestrials from the star system The Pleiades. The Pleiadian culture is ancient and was 'seeded' from another universe of love long before Earth was created....The Pleiadians are now here as ambassadors from another universe to help Earth through her difficult transition from the third dimension to the fourth dimension and to assist each of us in our personal endeavors of awakening, remembering and knowing."

Putative Pleiadians have been around since the first flying saucer stories started circulating fifty years ago. Their intimacy with earthlings is now taken for granted by all dedicated New Agers.

SUNSITE

**http://sunsite.unc.edu/pub/academic/medicine/
alternative-healthcare/**

This is the massive collection of articles on many different
subjects, maintained by the University of North Carolina,
that first got me seriously thinking about the Internet.

One of the unique things that Sunsite has done is to store and
catalog the discussions in various listservs and newsgroups. This is
very convenient, since if you want to look up a particular topic, you
can see what people were saying about it informally for years back.

I like this because although I do appreciate the nuggets of information contained in such discussions, I just hate to subscribe to
these things. They are usually such a waste of time. It doesn't matter whether you're discussing prostate cancer, UFOs, or classical
archeology, people rarely seem to stick to the point. They make
friends and enemies, chat about their lovers and spouses, and generally waste other people's time. Finally, it always turns out that
there are three loudmouths who have to dominate the whole conversation. At first they are allies, but soon they become raging enemies. "Flames" ensue, people demand that other people get
thrown off the group, and sometimes they are. Surefire topics
to ruin any listserv are (1) vaccinations; (2) animal rights; and

(3) vegetarianism. Yet, occasionally, something of interest does pass through these on-going discussions. So how do you find the gems among all this annoying verbiage? One way is to frequent Sunsite at the University of North Carolina. Basically, the good librarians at Sunsite have collected the day-to-day banter on a number of alternative medical topics, and organized them more or less by subject matter. "This collection of files represents ten years worth of gleanings from Usenet newsgroups, Internet mailing lists, gopher, ftp and WWW sites and FidoNet discussion forums." They suggest that you retrieve the INDEX file for a recursive listing of all directories and their contents.

Some of this is ancient, but still useful. The table of contents will give you some idea of the scope of this monster site:

Acupuncture	Diet and Nutritional Therapy	Music Therapy	Quackery
Addiction and Abuse		Native American Healing Traditions	Reflexology
Alexander Technique	Energy/Vibrational Medicine	Naturopathic Medicine	Reiki
Amma Therapy	EthnoMedical Links		Resonance Therapy
Apitherapy	Environmental Medicine	Neural Tissue Testing	Rolfing
Applied Kinesiology	Essence Therapy	Neuro Linguistic Programing	Shamanism
Aromatherapy	Feldenkrais Method		Shiatsu
Ayurvedic Medicine	Flower Remedies	Nootropic Pharmacology	Somatics
Biofeedback	Gesundheit! Institute	Nutritional Healing	Stress Management
Bio Oxidative Medicine	Hellerwork	Ortho-Bionomy	Sufi Healing
Body Mind Medicine	Herbal Medicine	Osteopathy	Tai Chi (Tai Ji)
Cancer Therapies	Holistic Medicine	Oxygen Therapy	Therapeutic Humor
Chelation Therapy	Homeopathy	Physical Therapy	Traditional Chinese Medicine
Chiropractic	Iridology	Preventive Medicine	Vegetarianism
Complementary Birthing Practices	Life Extension	Prolotherapy	Veterinary Medicine
Cryogenic Medicine	Light Therapy	Podiatry	Vision Enhancement
Dentistry	Massage Therapy	Polarity Therapy	Wellness
	Meditation	Qigong	Yoga

What exactly will you find here? Well, I went looking through the crystal healing section. I found a plaintive plea from Rae, looking for information regarding Amber. "What folklore is associated with this stone—good/bad. Would the intensity of the stone change with lack of impurities (insects, etc) trapped within it, as opposed to a clear stone?"

The answer she got back from another participant was actually "a leaflet purchased at Marie Laveau's House of Voodoo on the Rue Bourbon in New Orleans. Amber, according to the House of Voodoo "eases stress, improves memory, overcomes depression and helps the body to heal itself."

Or perhaps you are fascinated by ear candles? This is an alternative way of removing earwax by burning a candle right above the ear. How about this from someone named "bruceb" complaining bitterly that "the FDA pulled ear candles off the shelf because the wax might run down the candle into your ear."

Those crazy guys at FDA. Wherever do they get their ideas?

UNIV. OF TEXAS

http://www.sph.uth.tmc.edu/www/utsph/utcam/index.htm

This University of Texas site is funded by the Office of Alternative Medicine and represents the first time that a major university has undertaken the objective and dispassionate evaluation of some of the most controversial cancer treatments.

Until recently, there was virtually no reliable research going on into alternative cancer treatments. The medical authorities were confident in surgery, radiation and chemotherapy, and refused to perform such studies, as a waste of time and money. What limited tests were performed were sometimes marked by outright fraud.

How times have changed. First the OTA Report and then the formation of the OAM, with its Chantilly Report, changed the climate from total denial to a tentative acceptance of some such treatments.

Unable for summon the political will to do such research itself, the OAM has funded this project at the University of Texas. The goal of this project is three fold: to facilitate the scientific evaluations of biopharmacologic and herbal therapies as well as innovative approaches. • to establish a national network of alternative medicine practitioners, conventional practitioners, and researchers.

- to support the use of critical evaluation skills among alternative medicine practitioners and researchers.

Admittedly, most of this is a literature review so far. But scientific literature is also important, and during their first year, the Houston team has completed a systematic review of specific bio-pharmacologic and herbal products. They established an international network of alternative medicine researchers and practitioners. They also got their key advisory committees in place.

"During year two, our goal is to develop and initiate research protocols to evaluate specific treatments. But I think you will see that the level of scholarship is much higher than any previous academic discussion has been."

A lot of hopes are riding on this project. This Web page is a very straightforward presentation of what they have accomplished, including comprehensive reviews of the work of pioneer researchers such as Stanislaw R. Burzynski and Gaston Naessens.

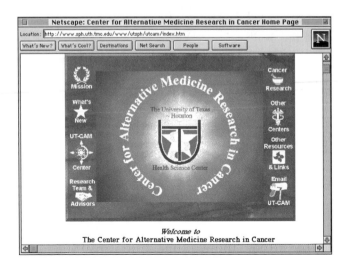

THORNE
RESEARCH

http://www.thorne.com

This would be just another commercial site,
albeit a particularly attractive one, if it weren't for their serious
effort to scientifically document the products they sell.

Thorne Research sells supplements. They have also done a lot of hard work, locating the most essential scientific articles that researchers are talking about or are relying on for their medical needs.

This site contains valuable scientific abstracts of articles on the following products and conditions: Acetyl-L-carnitine • Benign Prostatic Hypertrophy • Coenzyme Q10, Taurine, Crataegus • N-Acetylcysteine • DHEA (Dehydroepiandrosterone) • Ginkgo biloba • Glucosamine Sulfate • L-Glutamine • Green Tea Extract • Melatonin • Oligomeric Proanthocyanidins (Pycnogenols) • Pantethine • Pectin • Phosphatidylserine • Quercitin • Silymarin, Turmeric and Artichoke • Squalene • Vitamin A

For instance, Thorne has located and reprinted 12 key abstracts on pycnogenols, a grape seed extract that is highly touted by some proponents. If you search for "pycnogenol" in the government's excellent PubMed (my current favorite search engine; access is via http://www4.ncbi.nlm.nih.gov/PubMed/) you will come up with only four citations, none of which, for various reasons, overlaps with the Thorne compilation.

So if you are seriously interested in what is really known about one of the supplements listed above, Thorne's research is deep and very useful. Most of it dates from 1995 or so, and needs to be supplemented by recourse to the standard databases.

It is said that the field of food supplements is rife with shoddy practices. Thorne provides Net-izens with a valuable service and the data to make up their own minds.

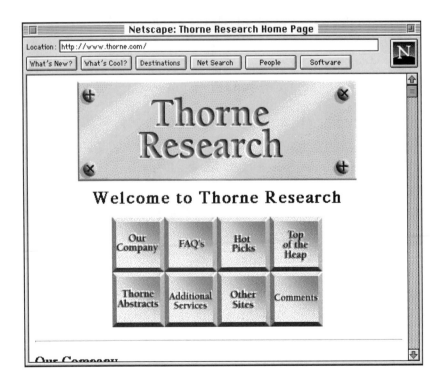

UPLEDGER INSTITUTE

http://www.upledger.com

"Site unseen," you might think this was just another
physical therapy clinic. You would be wrong.
The Upledger Institute is something special, a phenomenon,
with thousands of adherents around the world.

John Upledger, DO, founder of the Upledger Institute, developed
Cranio-Sacral Therapy (CST) and Somato-Emotional Release (SER).

John is an osteopath with a fairly orthodox medical background.
After 12 years in general practice in Florida, he accepted a faculty
position as a clinical researcher in the Department of Biomech-
anics at Michigan State University's College of Osteopathic Medicine. During the following eight years at Michigan State, he conducted research in the areas of osteopathic manipulation,
acupuncture, Kirlian photography, and the craniosacral system.

Actually, that hardly describes the revelation that came over him
when he became convinced that the spinal fluid actually moves
with a pulse-like motion. (I'm simplifying, of course.) The implications of this turned out to be vast for many areas of medicine.

In 1985, he founded The Upledger Institute in Palm Beach

Gardens, Florida, as a healthcare continuing education center and clinic. John continues to conduct research, teach and maintain a private practice there. I have been deeply impressed by the seriousness, dedication and intelligence of the cranio-sacral professionals. Upledger has built a large movement. He is a visionary in the field of medicine.

The Institute specializes in treating brain and spinal cord dysfunction; learning disabilities; infant to preschool evaluation; therapist rejuvenation; and post-traumatic stress disorder. They also offer instruction to the general public on how to relieve headaches, reduce stress, control pain, and promote relaxation.

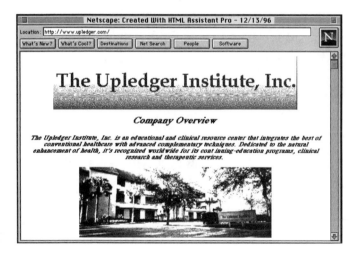

In their own words: "The Upledger Institute, Inc. is an educational and clinical resource center that integrates the best of conventional healthcare with advanced complementary techniques. Dedicated to the natural enhancement of health, it is highly regarded worldwide for its continuing-education programs, clinical research and therapeutic services."

URINE THERAPY

http://www.radiant-living.com/urine.htm

One of the wildest ideas in alternative medicine: drink your own urine for health.

That's right. Urine therapy. Or as they say at this site, Ur-Own Therapy. If you are new to this field, you may think I'm joking, but believe me these people are quite serious. Personally, I find the whole topic, er, distasteful. However, it is surprising how many people can bring themselves to down a hot toddy of bodily wastes.

There are whole books devoted to ecstatic expositions of the topic, such as the classic "The Water of Life, A Treatise On Urine Therapy" by J.W. Armstrong or the more recent "Your Own Perfect Medicine" by Martha M. Christy.

Allegedly, use of urine as medicine goes back to the Bible. But so does stoning women who wear red dresses. One good thing I can say about urine therapy: the price is certainly right. Also, you don't have to drive halfway across town to find a pharmacy open in the middle of the night. You are your own drug store.

I don't know if there is any medical value to this idea or not, but I find the rhetoric of urine therapy rather comical. They call urine an "elixir," which cures the common cold, rheumatism, arthritis, mucus colitis, obesity, prostate trouble, pyorrhea and many other disorders and diseases.

I did know one person with AIDS, a sensible fellow who worked for a major pharmaceutical company by day, but drank deeply of this topic by night. He claimed to have gotten rid of one Kaposi sarcoma lesion (a malignancy associated with AIDS) on the top of his palate in this way. Later, however, the treatment stopped working and the poor guy died.

Later on, I asked Stanislaw R. Burzynski, MD, PhD, what he thought about this sort of therapy. Dr. Burzynski is the Houston physician and drug developer, whose antineoplaston agents were themselves originally derived from human urine. Burzynski's comments were interesting. He in no way dismissed the possibility that ingesting urine might be beneficial in some instances, since urine normally contains growth inhibiting factors (such as his own antineoplastons). However, he also sensibly cautioned that urine could contain growth-promoting factors as well. So there was a risk for cancer patients in following this route.

This urine therapy site is rather inelegant, but it certainly contains some hard-to-find information. They invite you to email them at "clinic-urine@radiant-living.com," if you want to find out more about this sort of therapy.

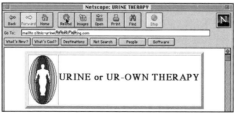

ANDREW WEIL

http://cgi.pathfinder.com/drweil

ASK DR. WEIL

This is probably the most popular alt.med.site on the Web, and with good reason. Andrew Weil is justly famous as a spokesperson for integrative medicine. He is well-educated, smart and good looking, too.

Plenty of people would love to have Dr. Weil for their doctor. So far Scottish scientists have been unable to clone him, but Time-Warner has done the next best thing: made him available on the Internet.

The site itself is predictably jazzy and fun. His popular approach pays off. He receives over one million hits per month, making this one of the most popular sites on the Net.

By and large, Dr. Weil is well tuned to his audience. He does not condescend to them, even when the question is about something as basic as peanut butter and jelly sandwiches. His advice is "progressive mainstream." Go ahead and eat p&j sandwiches, he says. But make it with whole wheat bread, almond butter (to avoid cancer-causing aflatoxins, he explains), and use unsugared jellies or jams. He manages to avoid purism in a field that is rife with it.

Sometimes Dr. Weil does seem to shoot from the hip, and to summarily dismiss some treatments that may have merit. But usually I find his advice sensible and generous towards other practitioners. About the popular book "Arthritis Cure," for instance, he avoids the cheap shots that abound in academia, and writes, "My view is that the program is worth trying. There's no risk of harm, and at minimum, you'll learn some things about incorporating a healthy diet and exercise routine into your life." Well put.

This site is an excellent introduction to alternative medicine—or integrative, as he prefers. Weil is a born leader and genuine teacher. He has a well deserved following of people who read his books, cram his seminars, watch his TV shows and now flock to his page. It is characteristic of his charisma that some devoted fans have even adopted "Ask Dr. Weil" as their own home page. His Santa Claus face is the first thing they see in the morning and the last thing they see at night.

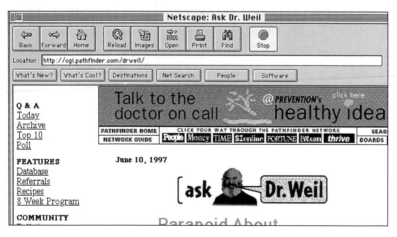

WELLNESS WEB

http://www.wellweb.com/

Originating in Villanova, Pennsylvania, the Wellness Web
is an extraordinary site. It has been rated one of the
Top 100 Web Sites of All Time! and according to Net Magazine,
"one of the top five in the world in the health category."

I can see why. The site is divided into three broad categories on complementary medicine, conventional medicine and nutrition/fitness.

Here's what they say about themselves:
> "WellnessWeb is a collaboration of patients, healthcare professionals, and other caregivers. Our mission is help you find the best and most appropriate medical information and support available.

You'll find information here about a wide variety of useful topics: clinical trials, community health, drug dosages and compliance, treatment options and research, how to select a physician, dozens of particular illnesses and conditions, tips for a healthy lifestyle, alternative/complementary treatment options, and much, much more.

"We think patients-consumers should have more input into the delivery and future of healthcare," they write. "We're trying to put the HEART back in health care, and hope you'll join us by making WellnessWeb a hub of activity."

A lot of sites purport to speak for patients. But the WellnessWeb was actually founded by patients who discovered just how difficult it was to become well enough informed to communicate with their doctors.They created a place to meet and exchange information such as could never exist without the Internet.

I consider this a very important site. That is because it is one of the few places where the advocates of alternative/complementary treatments and the "quackbusters" (professional denigraters) actually talk to each other. There was a very illuminating exchange of information—mostly negative—about the ubiquitous Dead Doctors Don't Lie tape (i.e., colloidal minerals).

That said, a lot of medical professionals hang out at the WellnessWeb and the alternative information that is offered sometimes verges on pontification.

WellnessWeb is struggling with the issue of making the Internet pay for a non-profit educational process. Their particular solution is to accept some paid advertising. "Educational grants give us absolute editorial control," they write. "For sponsorships, we may create specific client oriented pages within WellnessWeb. These pages will be clearly identified with a legend to the effect that 'this page is sponsored by....' When we link WellnessWeb to external sites of sponsorship clients, we will note to the effect that the link will take you to the site of a sponsor of WellnessWeb."

We wish them the best in this endeavor. As we all know, however, advertising can become the tail that wags the dog. That is why I favor independent, non-commercial sites. These sites may be wrong or foolish, but it won't be because someone paid them to be so.

Wellness Web is an excellent site, well worth a visit, especially if you are a patient perplexed about your medical care.

WOUND CARE INSTITUTE

http://www.wound.com/index.html

The authors of this site may be surprised to find themselves in a book about 'alternative medicine.' But serious innovators often find strange bedfellows with alt.med. advocates when their treatments try to defy the rules of economics.

Over the years, I have found myself drawn to those special situations in which unconventional treatments arise within orthodox medical institutions. Sometimes, important new discoveries are just not readily accepted, despite their intrinsic merit. These situations may or may not be "alternative" medicine. Who cares—as long as they are more effective and/or less harmful than competing therapies.

This "Wound Care Institute" site embodies such a situation. This is the group practice of two doctors, Ronald Scott and Jeffrey Stone, who run the Wound Care Clinic of North Texas, in the Institute for Exercise & Environmental Medicine at Presbyterian Hospital of Dallas. Essentially, they are using an accepted medical technique—hyperbaric oxygen—for unconventional purposes. Hyperbaric oxygen is conventional for the treatment of air or gas embolism; decompression sickness (the "bends") and carbon monoxide poisoning. But it is highly experimental for a lot of other conditions, including problematic non-healing wounds. (One might compare EDTA Chelation, which is standard for lead poisoning but controversial for cardiovascular disease.)

The Lone Star scientists use a variety of techniques for the management of persistent wounds, including:

Advanced Wound Dressings • Hyperbaric (High-pressure) Oxygen Treatment • Growth Factors • Antibiotic Therapy • Conventional Wound Dressings • Nutrition Counseling • Education/Prevention • Surgery • Physical Therapy • Protective Footwear

Pre-eminent among the situations they treat, however, are wounds that will not heal. Even the ancient Greeks knew how maddening such problems could be. Sophocles wrote a play, Philoctetes, based around this medical problem.

An extraordinary five million Americans now suffer from chronic open sores which can become seriously infected, gangrenous or even require amputation. In fact, we read here that nearly 70 percent of medical amputations result from the complications of chronic wounds. Usually, these wounds have been treated with topical ointments, antibiotics and other remedies which only touch the surface of the problem.

Although standard medical applications may relieve pain and cause temporary improvements, doctors at the Wound Care Clinic of North Texas say that permanent healing of chronic wounds will not occur until the treatment takes aim at the fundamental source of the problem. The kinds of wounds they specialize in include:

Diabetic Skin Sores • Pressure Sores • Vessel Disease Wounds • Surgery Wound Breakdown • Spinal Injury Wounds • Chemical Wounds

The site itself is straightforward and rather attractive. When I find a site like this it makes the hundreds of hours spent searching the Web seem worthwhile. I think about how much hope it could give to the person facing a limb amputation who comes across a site like this and finds fresh hope.

Once again, you see the power of the Internet at its very best.

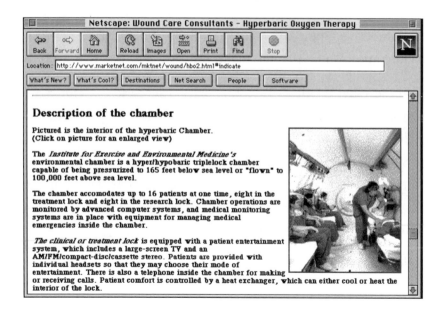

WORLDWIDE WELLNESS

http://www.wholeliving.com

A site of incredible richness and diversity.
There is also exceptional color artwork here that simply
does not reproduce in black and white.

Their motto is "Show Up....Pay Attention....Tell Truth....Stay Open to Outcome." Would that all health professionals had that attitude!

What they say: "WorldWide Wellness: Internet Resources for Whole Living, is a comprehensive database of alternative and wholistic health information and resources. WorldWide Wellness utilizes Intermedia Synergy to unite the online world with the wholistic community. Access our growing Professional Directory of Wholistic Goods and Services and read articles from the forefront of mind/body/spirit research."

Under "articles" you will find some very provocative thinking on matters of health and holism:

Mindfulness in the Classroom
Discover Your Quiet Mind: A Technology for the 90s
Does Anybody Really Know What Time It Is?

In addition, there is an incredible list of articles which form a kind of primer of alternative medical techniques:

Universal Aspects of Healing
Holistic Medicine
First Do No Harm
The Return of the Green Man
Rolfing® and Stiff, Achy Muscles
Hands, Hearts, Intentions
Shamanism and the Spirit World
Miracle of Magnetics
Chiropractic: End Pain Naturally
Homeopathy: The Safer Medicines
The Air You Breathe
The Secret to Mind is No-Mind
Agnihotra: Healing Ash, Pyramids and Cow Manure
Long Live the Men's Movement!
Depression: A Pathway Home to the Self
Should You Consider a Feminist Therapist?
Colonics: Using Water to De-Stress the Body = Relief
AIT: Treatment for Attention Deficit and Other Learning Disorders
Feldenkrais®
Zen Shiatsu
Traditional Chinese Medicine
Expresssive and Experiential Psychotherapies
Choosing a Holistic Dentist
Massage for Women Recovering from Abuse
The Emotional Body: An Interview with Candace Pert, PhD
Look Great, Feel Great, Chew Great

This list is emblematic of alternative medicine as a whole. It is a mixture of profound thoughts, medical breakthroughs, and just a tad of New Age nonsense. Yet even the nonsense may contain some nuggets of value. Some things in alternative medicine are fairly well documented procedures whose main crime is that they can't make much money for the pharmaceutical industry. Others are time-tested folk techniques which are probably harmless and possibly beneficial. The healing power of cow manure, urine therapy and the subtle emanations of crystals seems weird. But without good medical research, who is to say?

CONCLUSION

Once upon a time, if you got sick, your doctor prescribed a medicine, and you either got better or you suffered. But you didn't question. It was unheard of to seriously doubt your own doctor.

Today, thanks to the Net, you have instant access to a vast and growing trove of material on almost every medical topic. This is available day and night in various gradations of technical complexity. If you are a seasoned Netizen, it is often your doctor who winds up questioning *you* about new treatments.

As this book has hopefully demonstrated, the Net gives you access to breathtaking new ideas, scorned scientific geniuses, astonishing new methods. It also is a fertile breeding ground for the dubious proposition, the self-serving fraud, and even a few old-fashioned back-of-the-wagon quacks. To tell the difference takes discernment. I have written this book in the hope that it will not only point you to worthy sites but convey a way of looking at alternative medicine that is open-minded yet critical, serious yet amused.

Most of all, I want us to be free to educate ourselves and make up our own minds. There are rumblings of censoring the Net in order to "protect" the hapless victims of quackery. Let's resist censorship in any guise. All new ideas should be given exposure, because amidst them all are undoubtedly some of tremendous potential. The answer is to hone our own critical faculties, to entertain the radically new while retaining our innate common sense. —R.W.M.

INDEX

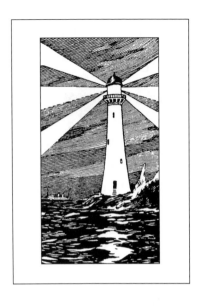

HEALING CHOICES REPORT SERVICE

Reports for Individuals
with Cancer
Personally researched
and written
by Ralph W. Moss, Ph.D.

Consulting an expert can be helpful to you in many ways. If you or someone you love has cancer, you probably have many questions about alternative treatment options. You want to educate yourself in order to make informed decisions, and you don't want to waste time.

Your Healing Choices report by Ralph W. Moss, Ph.D., will provide you with objective, detailed information on the most promising alternative methods and practitioners for your particular type of cancer. Alternative cancer therapies are difficult to evaluate. There are hundreds of treatments and many present conflicting claims. Your Healing Choices report will give you detailed and prioritized information on practitioners and treatments that he feels are the most valid and relevant to your situation.

Please call Anne Beattie, coordinator, at 1-718-636-4433 to request a Healing Choices packet, which contains a questionnaire. When you send or fax back that questionnaire, you will be informed when to expect your completed report.

Other books by Ralph W. Moss, Ph.D. from Equinox Press

The Cancer Industry: The Classic Exposé on the Cancer Establishment

This book shows why the billion dollar war on cancer is going nowhere. It details how drug companies influence cancer policy, how major industries keep the emphasis away from prevention, how the establishment maintains a blacklist of unconventional practitioners, and how the government has collaborated in the suppression of new ideas.

$16.95   528 pp. trade paperback

Cancer Therapy: The Independent Consumer's Guide to Non-Toxic Treatment & Prevention

You want the full story on non-toxic treatment and prevention, and that's exactly what this landmark book delivers. Cancer Therapy is a must for cancer patients and their families who want: practical information on the most promising, non-toxic treatments; scientific evidence in readable language; well documented resource lists and medical references. Author Ralph W. Moss, Ph.D. has been called "possibly the best science writer in our midst" and "a revolutionary in the war on cancer."

$19.95 528 pp trade paperback

Questioning Chemotherapy

Finally, a powerful and intelligent critique of chemotherapy! This up-to-date book from acclaimed medical writer Ralph W. Moss, Ph.D. probes the scientific and statistical evidence to reveal the shocking truth: chemotherapy is inappropriate, ineffective and, in fact, dangerous for most of the people who receive it. Yet up to 600,000 Americans every year get chemo at their doctor's recommendation. "A masterpiece of global importance in the history of medicine."—Hans Nieper, MD, Past Pres., German Society of Oncology

$19.95 214 pp trade paperback